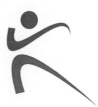

Fit Kids

7–17 YEARS

THE PERFECT START TO A HEALTHY LIFE

First published in Great Britain in 2016 by:

BX Plans Ltd
Remus House
Coltsfoot Drive
Peterborough
PE2 9BF
United Kingdom

Contents

The Charts

Introduction

I magine a fitness plan that comprises just five elements. Imagine a fitness plan that takes just 11 minutes of your time in a day. Imagine a fitness plan that needs no extra equipment, no visits to the gym, but helps you to lead a more active, healthy life. The BX fitness plans are a simple-to-use but progressive series of exercises that help develop strength, flexibility and aerobic fitness for people of all ages and abilities.

These plans are not a new fad, they have a proven track record and have been tested in the most challenging of spheres.The BX fitness plans were first developed by the Royal Canadian Air Force (RCAF) in the 1950s. 5BX – five basic exercises – was the brainchild of Bill Orban, who was tasked with developing a fitness plan for the pilots of the RCAF, many of whom were considered unfit to fly at the time.

The plans met two criteria: they were time efficient – just 11 minutes – and they required no additional equipment. Orban devised a plan that was progressive and effective and more than 65 years on, those plans are as relevant today as they were in the 1950s.

The founder of BX fitness plans first discovered 5BX in the 1970s and then re-discovered these exercises after a 40 year break. Although four decades older, he was soon on his way to a healthier and more active life. His goal now is to make the BXPlans relevant to all generations. The premise: simple exercises that can be done anywhere and only take 11 minutes and can be used by adults and children. The plans get you into an exercise routine, which is the foundation of a healthy, active life.

BX fitness programmes offer an easy way to get fit and, through their progressive nature, guide you to reach your fitness potential. In this book, we have adapted the 5BX fitness programme to make it both relevant and simple to implement, so whether you are a parent, carer, teacher, coach or teaching assistant, you will have the resources to offer a fun-filled, practical route to helping children live an active and healthy lifestyle.

This book is designed to complement the BX fitness exercise charts, giving you some of the science behind health and fitness and offering additional exercises and activities to help you deliver a healthy, active lifestyle through the child's formal school curriculum. There are no hard and fast rules in the book, but the ideas contained within can be adapted to suit children from school year 3-6. Chapters 8-10 contain ideas that will help families to undertake more active lives. Our ultimate aim? Fit schools and fit families.

Chapter One

Why exercise is important

Understanding why exercise matters is the first step in developing a life-long habit. The link between good physical and mental health and regular exercise is one that every child should recognise and understand from an early age. Teaching children about the importance of regular exercise should be the priority of parents/carers in the home environment and teachers via both the formal and informal curriculum.

In a society where a third of all 10-11 year olds are either obese or overweight (Public Health England), encouraging children to get active and teaching them about the importance of exercise and healthy eating is just one step towards reversing the obesity crisis that is fast becoming a public health epidemic. Not enough physical activity, too much access to sugary foods and drinks and an increasingly sedentary lifestyle has led us to a place where the younger generation are likely to have a lower life expectancy than their parents for the first time in history.

Here is the science: physical inactivity is a major risk factor for developing coronary artery disease. It also increases the risk of stroke and such other major cardiovascular risk factors such as obesity, high blood pressure, low HDL ("good") cholesterol and diabetes. Just like in adults, increased physical activity in children has been associated with an increasing life expectancy and decreased risk of developing cardiovascular disease in later life.

Small measures can address the problems, just a small amount of extra activity a day can make a huge difference to a child's health. Just 11/12 minutes of exercise a day can improve a child's heart and lung capacity; increase their circulation, balance and coordination; help them develop stronger muscles and bones; and improve their psychological well-being.

Being active – five BIG benefits

- Helps children develop strong bones and muscles
- Improves children's cardiovascular (heart and lungs) system
- Reduces the risk of some chronic diseases in later life
- Reduces body fat and helps them feel good about themselves
- Improves social development and reduces anxiety and stress

Activity

Organise a game of 'it' in the playground. After the game, ask the children to write down three words that describe how they felt during the course of the game. Create a mood board using vibrant colours to reflect their feelings and emotions resulting from exercise.

Changing the mindset

When we mention exercise, as adults, we tend to think about working out in the gym, grinding out the miles on a run, lifting weights or attending a fitness class. For many adults, this is something we SHOULD do, rather than something we WANT to do. It is at this point that we must leave those negative thoughts behind and see things through a child's eyes.

Exercise for children means playing and being physically active. While the underlying aim is to increase the child's activity levels, the means for doing that have to be fun and enjoyable. Through the pages of this book and the BX fitness plan, you will be able to provide the children in your care with meaningful activities that will get them active and help form a life-long fitness habit.

Within children's activity, be it formal lessons or informal 'play', three main fitness elements will always be running through children's activities. These are endurance, strength and flexibility. Think about a child's day. In the playground he or she might run away from the person who is 'it (endurance); the child might swing from a bar or hang from a railing (strength); and bending to tie shoe-laces or curling up in an unfeasibly tight ball to listen to a story being read are both forms of flexibility.

Through BX Fitness plans we will help your children, and the children in your care, to develop these three aspects of fitness and make movement and activity a fun part of every day.

Chapter 2

What happens when we exercise?

All sorts of changes happen when we exercise. We get a red face, we sweat, our heart pounds, our lungs pump and we feel brighter and more alert.

When we first exercise, some of these things can be alarming, so let's take a whistle-stop tour of the body and find out just what is going on.

Breathing heavily

When we exercise, our muscles are called into action. To power the muscles, the body needs energy, which is stored in the body in the form of a sugar called **glycogen** and another energy source called **adenosine triphosphate** (ATP). When these energy sources run out, the body asks for more oxygen to be delivered, which will provide more ATP. Sometimes we can need up to 15 times more oxygen when we exercise. This is why we breathe heavier when we exercise.

Activity

March or jog on the spot for 30 seconds. Take a rest and while you are resting listen to how your breathing has changed. Now march or jog on the spot for 2 minutes. During your rest, see if you are breathing harder this time. Now run as quickly as you can on the spot for 30 seconds. How do you feel. Can you draw a chart that shows the relationship between how hard you worked and your breathing rate.

Face changes colour

As we work harder during a physical activity, our body, like any machine, produces heat and needs to cool down. To do this, the blood vessels in the skin dilate (get wider) which means more blood flows to the surface of the body, just under the skin. As the blood is nearer the air, it will gradually cool, but the skin will have turned red because there is more blood at the body's surface. This is particularly true in the skin's surface on the face.

Sweating

When we exercise, our sweat glands get to work. The **eccrine glands**' job is to control the body's temperature so the glands produce perspiration – a mixture of water, salt and small amounts of electrolytes. These are transported directly to the skin's surface and, as the sweat evaporates into the air, so your body temperature drops. This perspiration is odourless.

The **apocrine glands** produce sweat on the scalp, groin and armpits. This is a fattier sweat and is often produced at times of emotional stress as well as physical stress. For example, when waiting for an important match to begin or before the start of a race. This sweat can result in odour when bacteria on the skin starts to break the sweat down.

As we lose moisture through sweating, it is important that we drink plenty of water to replace the moisture.

Getting 'stitch'

Like any muscle, the **diaphragm** can grow tired during exercise. The diaphragm is very involved in pumping more oxygen to the body, so as we breath more heavily, the diaphragm is under enormous pressure. If the diaphragm gets tired, it can spasm. This is the sensation that we know as 'stitch', when we get a sudden sharp pain in our side. Deep breathing and stretching can alleviate the discomfort and as we get fitter, so the chance of stitch lessens.

Heart pumping faster

As you exercise, your body needs blood to be pumped around it faster. This blood carries the extra oxygen that is required by the muscles. At the centre of this is the heart – the work station of the body. When you are exercising, you will feel your heart gradually beating faster as it pumps the blood through the network of arteries, veins and capillaries. As you get fitter, so your heart will be able to cope with the demands better and so it doesn't have to pump so hard.

Chapter 3

Fitness in the curriculum and beyond

For children, physical activity needs to be fun and enjoyable. The BX plans can be incorporated into the school day at any time and anywhere, they can be used to re-energise children part way through a sedentary lesson or they can be an intrinsic part of the curriculum linked to a range of subjects in a variety of exciting ways.

Here are just a few examples of ways the fitness plan can be incorporated into the school day.

1 As part of assembly or at the start of the school day

In the assembly hall, the sports hall or, on a fine day, on the school playing field, lead a whole school fitness session. Everyone can get involved, from the youngest pupil to the most senior teacher. This is an energising and sociable way to start the school day. There will be a buzz about the school for the rest of the day.

2 As a mid–morning energiser

The class has been sitting down for the last half an hour, struggling with a particularly tricky mathematics problem. Take a few minutes to get everyone on their feet, doing part of the fitness plan. Just three minutes of activity will re-energise the children, ensuring that they are breathing deeper and increasing the flow of oxygen around their body. Repeat this at different times of the day until the whole plan has been completed.

3 As part of a lesson

This is where teachers can demonstrate their vast ability to make lessons fun and relevant. Include exercises in the main curriculum: as the basis for a science experiment; as an art project; the subject of a poem; a design and technology project. Ask the children to write a report on the exercises for the school newspaper; even put the exercises to music. The 5BX fitness plan could be the central premise behind a cross-curricular project.

4 As a charity fundraiser

Can the 5BX fitness plan be the focus of a charity fundraiser – challenge the children to do the exercises every day for a month in aid of charity. Again, this can be a whole school challenge and is a simple way to help the children form a life-long exercise habit.

5 As an opportunity to develop leadership skills

Young children can take the lead on the fitness programme as a way to develop and demonstrate leadership skills. The Year 6 pupils could lead groups of younger children through the exercises, either at break time or during physical education sessions. The plans are easy to follow and will provide a great opportunity for young leaders to develop communication skills.

6 As a community project

If your school has a link with an old people's home or a care centre, this could be a great opportunity for your pupils to help get others active. Once your pupils have mastered all the moves themselves and can demonstrate how to do each exercise, then they can take that knowledge into the wider community. Working with people in care centres is a great way for the children to develop many life-long skills and qualities: communication, organisation, empathy and care. It will also help spread the habit of regular exercise to the wider community.

7 As a social activity

Getting together as a class, a year group or a whole school to take part in a daily exercise routine is a great way to get children mixing. Maybe the session can be organised so children work with other year groups or with pupils they do not normally mix with. There is also the possibility that parents and children of pre-school age can come into the sessions and join in – again, a great opportunity to encourage activity and reinforce its importance to the wider community.

Chapter 4

Other activities

Whilst BX fitness plans are the basis for a life-long exercise habit, adding other formal and informal activities into the children's daily activities will add excitement, inspiration and motivation.

In addition, as the children progress with the fitness plan, they will find they are capable of running for longer, moving with greater ease and balance and generally feel more lively. Now they need somewhere for all that energy to go.

Here are some activities that children can get involved in during the school day.

Informal play

Hide and seek

One of the most popular games, involving people running away to hide and others running around to find them. Sometimes there is a 'home base' to get to, sometimes you just wait to be found.

Jump rope or Double Dutch

Using a long rope, with a person at each end turning the rope, people take turns at jumping/skipping. This can be done with one person jumping or a number of people jumping in at the same time. The activity is often performed in time to a rhyme.

Red Light, Green Light

One person is the traffic light, the other players stand some way back from them. When the traffic light faces the group of players, he or she says, "Red Light" and everyone must freeze. The traffic light turns his or her back and says, "Green Light", and the group moves to try and get as close as possible to the traffic light. The traffic light turns quickly, saying "Red Light". Anyone who is spotted moving when it is "Red Light" goes back to the starting position. The first person to tag the traffic light wins.

'It' or 'tag'

One person or a team are designated 'it' and their job is to try and tag everyone. If tagged, players might be sent to a holding pen until the last person is caught.

More formal play

Parachute

- This game involves a large round parachute or other light fabric, preferably with handles. People hold the edge of the parachute all around the edges. Players ruffle the parachute up and down, until it is rippling high enough for everyone to run underneath it and sit inside the parachute. Players can also place light objects such as bean bags in the centre of the parachute and wave the 'chute up and down to see how high the bean bag will jump. There are countless variations on this game and, while it is a good idea to have an adult supervisor, leaving the children to explore activities will stimulate their imagination and creativity.

Hare and Hounds

One or two children are chosen to be 'hounds'. Every other child wears a bib and is a 'hare'. The playing boundary is decided so players can not go 'Out of Bounds'. The hounds have to try to catch the hares; if they do, the hare takes off their bibs and become hounds as well. The last hare to be caught is the winner.

Bench ball

The game involves two teams, two benches – which are set out at either end of a designated area – a ball, and some bibs. Each team nominates one player to stand on the bench in their half of the area (the goalkeeper). The rest of the players arrange themselves anywhere in their half (apart from the bench). The game starts when the teacher throws the ball into the centre of the court, and any player can try to gain possession.

The aim of the game is to score goals by passing the ball around your team in order to pass it back to your goalkeeper on the bench. Each team has to make five passes before getting the ball to their keeper. If the ball is dropped or the opposition gain possession, then the count starts again.

When a goal is scored the opposition restarts with a throw from the goalkeeper.

Values of informal play

- Because the structure is informal, players use their interpersonal skills by choosing sides and organising the rules.

- Players take responsibility for resolving disputes and collaborating with peers so the game can continue.

- There is less stress as there is no external pressure to win/score points/ perform well.

- Problem solving, cooperation and improvisation are all skills used during informal play sessions.

Chapter 5

Fitness–based activities

The activities discussed in Chapter Four are very much play and game focused. This chapter looks at more fitness based activities that a class teacher or a teaching assistant can deliver that will help achieve specific fitness goals.

Aerobic activity

This can involve walking, jogging, running, sprinting, skipping, hopping or jumping. The aim is to raise the heart rate and get the oxygen travelling speedily around the body. This will increase the capacity of the heart and lungs. For adults, aerobic training would normally mean running on the treadmill or going for a power walk – for children, this needs to be fun and free-flowing, so the best way to get children working on their aerobic fitness is to incorporate movement into a game or fun activity.

One great way of improving cardiovascular or aerobic fitness and to engage children in a wider, educational task is to run an orienteering course. This is like a treasure hunt, with children following a map to find check points. The orienteering course can be as challenging or as simple as you want to make it, but the key thing is – it will get the children moving.

What is Orienteering

Orienteering is an exciting and challenging outdoor sport that exercises both mind and body. The aim is to navigate between control points marked on a map; as a competitive sport the challenge is to complete the course in the quickest time choosing your own best route; as a recreational activity, you can run or walk making progress at your own pace on the courses planned to suit you. This could be on the school playground, on the playing field or even in the school building. In the first instance the teacher should prepare easy to follow maps and set out the course but, over time, the children can draw maps for others in the group to follow.

Muscle strengthening

Gymnastics lessons are a great way to help children develop healthy and strong bones and muscles. The activities can range from simple roly-polys, which will help a child develop flexibility in his or her back to climbing bars and ropes, which will help their arm and leg muscles develop. A gym circuit is a good way to introduce children to a range of movement.

Setting up a gym circuit

Using a set of cards numbered 5-15, set out between 8-10 activity stations. These stations could include: jump rope, sit-ups, push-ups, star jumps, lunges, hopping from side to side, jumping over a low obstacle. The children start at one station and run to the centre of the room to collect a card, the value on the card is how many repetitions of each exercise they must do. They move around the stations in a clockwise direction.

Flexibility

Gymnastics is also a fantastic way to develop agility and flexibility. Encourage children to explore a whole range of movements by setting them challenges – can they spell their name by getting their bodies to make shapes of the alphabet for example?

Partner stretches is another way to get children exploring movement. In pairs, one child performs any bodily stretch, such as bending at the toes or reaching up high. The partner mirrors or copies the stretch. You can also use partners to increase stretches and encourage even greater mobility. One child performs a stretch and his or her partner gently moves the limbs to perform the stretch to a greater intensity. It is important that there is adult supervision during these exercises as young children can be vulnerable to injury, particularly if their body is going through a growth spurt.

Chapter Six

Checking progress

Through the BX Fitness Plan children will be able to recognise their own progress as they move through the levels of achievement. More exercises in the same amount of time indicates a growing reserve of aerobic fitness, strength and flexibility and children will be able to take pride in that.

There will also be the intrinsic knowledge that they are getting fitter. A child will feel more active and more able to exert energy and the changes in their body will be clear for their friends and family to see.

Greater agility and flexibility, an ability to run for longer without getting breathless, more strength in the arms, legs and core, higher energy levels, greater levels of self-confidence and a lowering of stress levels are all signs that a child is increasing his or her fitness levels. Children may also sleep more soundly at night and be more alert during the day.

There are also scientific means of charting a child's fitness and these can be incorporated very successfully into other areas of the school curriculum. Here are some examples:

Pulse rate

Your heart is a muscle that pumps blood around the body via the arteries. When we exercise, we call on the heart to provide more oxygen. Exercising the heart makes it bigger and stronger so that it doesn't have to work so hard to push the blood around the body. This means that as you get fitter, your heart rate will not need to pump as quickly to supply blood: each pump of the heart will send a large volume of blood charging around the body.

When we stop exercising, the heart rate returns to a resting heart rate and as a general rule, the lower our resting heart rate the fitter we are. So measuring a child's resting heart rate will indicate how fit that child is. We do this by measuring the pulse rate. This is the point where the artery is close to the skin's surface, normally at the wrist or neck. Get the children to work in pairs to help each other find and record pulse rate.

Activity

Show the class how to locate the pulse, either in the wrist or neck. Get the children to work in pairs. They take each other's pulse rate before exercising and record the figures. One child jogs on the spot for one minute. As soon as he or she has stopped jogging take the pulse again and record it. Now wait for one minute and record the pulse again, keep taking the pulse at minute intervals until the pulse rate is back to its original figure. As the children get fitter, so the pulse should return to the resting rate very soon after finishing an activity.

To calculate the pulse

Find the pulse, count for 30 seconds and then multiply that figure by two. This gives you beats per minute.

Tests to demonstrate muscular strength (upper body)

The Flexed Arm Hang is a test to measure upper body strength and endurance. Grab an overhead bar with arms bent and chin at bar level. Now hold that position for as long as possible. Repeat every two weeks and try to beat your time.

Test to demonstrate muscular strength (core/abdominals)

The curl-up is a type of sit-up

Children lie on their back with their legs up in the air at a 90-degree angle. Their hands are placed flat on the floor by their sides, and they curl (or crunch) up until their shoulder blades come off the floor. They complete as many repetitions as they can in a 30 second period. The more repetitions done in the time means a greater amount of muscle endurance.

Test to demonstrate flexibility

Sit and Reach Test

The sit and reach test measures the flexibility of the lower back and hamstring muscles. The test involves sitting on the floor with legs straight ahead, then reach as far forward as possible. Measure the distance the child's hands are from their toes or beyond their toes. Repeat the test every two weeks to chart progress.

Test to demonstrate aerobic fitness

Complete one mile (measured out in the playground or on the school playing field) and record your time. Repeat this every three weeks to see if you are getting fitter. As your aerobic capability increases, so your time should decrease. The mile can be walked, jogged or run.

Chapter Seven

Healthy Eating

The right nutrition is important for everyone, but especially for children as they need to put the right fuel into their bodies to help them develop and grow. Exercise and healthy eating go hand in hand – both are good for children, but together they are a dynamite combination. Like establishing good exercise habits early on in life, by establishing good eating habits, a child is more likely to develop a healthy eating habit later in life.

So what does healthy eating mean in practice? Here are our super six rules for healthy eating.

1 Children should enjoy their food

This will help establish positive attitudes towards food both as children and later in life. In the school setting, getting children interested in food early on will help them develop their interest in food and healthy eating.

2 Eat a balanced diet consisting of a mixture of different food groups

Foods contain different nutrients so children who eat a varied diet are more likely to be getting all the nutrients they need.

Activity

In art, get children to design and make a green grocers shop and see how many fruit and vegetables they can think of to stock their shelves.

3 Children and adults should be eating plenty of fruit and vegetables, raw, fresh, dried, canned and frozen are all ways of eating plenty of fruit and vegetables

4 **It is important that children eat energy-giving starchy foods such as bread, cereal, pasta, rice, couscous, potatoes and plantains**

They should also be eating at least one portion of protein with each meal – meat, fish, beans, lentils, soya for example.

5 **Try to avoid processed foods such as pastries, cakes, biscuits, crisps.**

These are high in calories but low in nutritional value. Some fats, in moderation, can be eaten as the body needs some essential fats to function well. Good fats, generally unsaturated fats, can be found in olive oil, oily fish and unsalted nuts.

6 **Cut down on additional sugar and salt.**

Sugar and salt are the bad guys when it comes to healthy eating. Not only does sugar rot children's teeth but it makes for all sorts of weight issues and it can create excessive moods swings as children have 'sugar highs' followed by dramatic lows. Salt just doesn't need to be added to food. It also has all sorts of impact upon health, causing high blood pressure in later life.

Activity

Working in groups, ask children to design a three-course meal that has the right balance of food stuffs in it. You could give a list of ingredients that they can select from or they can come up with ideas of their own. If you have the facilities, you could have a cooking class where the children make one or more parts of their menu.

The most important meal of the day?

Breakfast is important to top up children's energy stores for the morning's activities. Children who eat a healthy breakfast are less likely to snack on foods that are high in fat and/or sugar later on and tend to concentrate and perform better at school.

Chapter Eight

Getting family and friends into fitness

It is all well and good learning about healthy lifestyles through school, but what about when children go home? Wouldn't it be great if children were able to go home and spread the message about regular exercise to the rest of their family and friends?

By working together, schools and families can reinforce the messages about getting active and eating well. And by the same token, children might be able to change the way other members of their family live their lives.

Here are 10 ways this can be achieved.

1 Eat at the table together
Studies show families who have regular meals at the table with no distractions (such as television, tablets or computer games) are more likely to be a healthy weight and it makes for great sociable family time.

2 Include everyone in family activities
Get grandparents and children out walking the dog; encourage children to wash the car or mow the lawn; go for a family bike ride.

Doing these activities together will make it seem less as a chore or an organised exercise - it will just be fun.

3 Ban "sweetened" drinks from the home – persuade your children to drink water instead.
Fizzy drinks, fruit drinks, sports drinks, milky drinks with added sugar, and even 100 per cent fruit juice are high in calories. Children tend to drink fewer sweet drinks when they're not freely available in the home.

4 **Make sure the whole family eats breakfast every day – children who eat breakfast are less likely to overeat later in the day.**

If time is an issue, choose speedy yet healthy items such as peanut butter on wholemeal toast, or porridge and fruit.

5 **Agree as a family to decrease screen time – and put physical activity in its place.**

Turn the TV, computer and games consoles off, and instead get active as a family by walking, cycling, going to the park or playground, or swimming together.

6 **Get active on holiday – it's the perfect opportunity to get fit and have fun.**

You could try a specific activity-focused break, such as cycling or hiking, or choose a destination where you can do a variety of activities. Children generally love camping holidays. There's lots of scope for activity for children of all ages, from putting up the tent to nature hikes.

7 **Prepare more meals at home – it takes a little longer, but this way you can control what you put in food.**

You can read food labels, use healthier ingredients, and control how much sugar and salt you use.

8 **Have healthier takeaways – you don't have to give up takeaways completely, just make smarter choices.**

For instance, have mushy peas with your fish and chips and don't eat all the batter around the fish. Order lower-fat pizza toppings like vegetables, ham and prawns instead of salami and four-cheese. And with Indian takeaways, go for tomato-based sauces such as madras instead of cream-based kormas and masalas.

9 **Avoid over–sized portions**

Portion sizes have increased over the years and it's one of the reasons children become overweight. Start meals with small servings and let your child ask for more if they're still hungry. Avoid giving adult-sized plates to younger children – it can encourage them to eat too much.

10 **Walk for charity - doing regular charity walks is a great way for the whole family to get fit.**

Events are held across the country and are aimed at all ages, levels and abilities. Look for charity walks in your area.

Chapter Nine

Age appropriate activities

T his book has, hopefully, given you some good ideas to get you started on regular exercise sessions with the children in your care. Introducing exercise and activity as fun and linking it to as many parts of the school curriculum as possible is key to making physical activity a life-long habit, but, as with everything, there are other factors to consider.

One of these is the question of what children should be doing at each stage of their childhood. You know how it goes, you introduce the children to running and suddenly they all want to be Mo Farah. At what age do you encourage competition?

Here are some general guidelines:

Pre-school age

These tiny tots need play and exercise that helps them develop their motor skills – balance, movement, flexibility and coordination. Kicking or throwing a ball, playing tag or follow-my-leader, hopping, jumping, skipping, climbing small obstacles and learning to ride a bike (with stabilisers to begin) – basically any fun activity that gets them moving. Organised and team sports are not really appropriate at this age as the children will not recognise complex rules, getting the fundamental skills mastered is key.

School-age:

Ironically, when children become old enough to go to school, so their sedentary time tends to increase. Sitting at desks, doing homework, watching television and playing on the computer all adds to the time they spend sitting down. The challenge is for parents and teachers to find activities that will challenge and motivate them. From five onwards children can start getting involved in sports that they enjoy and can get success from – basketball, martial arts, swimming, cycling – and that will help develop motor skills further. It is at this point that children start to recognise if they are successful at a sport, so it is important that they find activities they enjoy and from which they gain an element of success and self confidence.

The danger at this age is to cram too many organised activities into the child's schedule. Don't forget to leave time for free play and exploration.

Fitness personalities

You only have to look at sports stars on television to recognise that certain personality types are attracted to certain sports and activities. The same is true of children. Personality types, genetics and athletic ability will all combine to determine whether a child is a team-sports player, an individual sports player (such as a swimmer or athlete) or more interested in recreation-type activities such as hiking, climbing or dancing.

You can divide children (and adults) into three very broad groups:

1 The non–athlete

This child may lack interest in sport or just consider themselves to have no athletic ability whatsoever. As a teacher or parent you need to give this child options that keep him or her active but do not destroy any self-confidence. Walking, dancing, orienteering, cycling are all activities that can be energetic without being competitive.

2 The causal athlete

This child wants to be active but is rarely the star player. The risk is that this child becomes discouraged whenever he or she is involved in a competitive environment. Pairing or teaming these children up with others of like ability is one answer to creating a good experience in a sporting setting.

3 The athlete

This child has a high level of physical ability and can turn his or hand to most sports. He or she should be encouraged to join clubs and commit to sports as they will need constant challenge to feed their energy and competitive levels.

FIT KIDS

The better you understand how different personality types view and approach exercise, activity and sport, the better you will be able to help each child find his or her place on the activity spectrum. Some children want to pursue excellence, others are happy to lead an active life, still others will need cajoling.

Whatever their needs, there is no reason why every child should not be physically active. A positive environment at school and at home is essential in achieving this.

Chapter 10

What can I do to get – and keep – the children in my care active?

As a teacher or as a parent/carer, you can help shape children's attitudes and behaviours toward physical activity and exercise. Introducing them to regular daily exercise in small amounts is a great place to start as it begins to develop a habit. As the children start to feel the benefits of the exercise, without knowing it, they will start to be more active themselves.

Below are seven key points to help you set a positive example.

- Set a positive example by leading an active lifestyle yourself. Talk about the activities you have done, tell funny stories abut things that have happened during your activity or exercise. If you take part in an event, share that with the children, bring in photos or reports.

- Make physical activity part of your daily classroom routine by taking time out of lessons to get the children stretching and moving. You can add movement into the curriculum in so many interesting ways. How about a nature walk around the school grounds or a treasure hunt as part of a geography lesson?

- Invest in equipment that encourages physical activity. Buy a selection of balls, beanbags, skipping ropes and hoops and keep them in an accessible place so the children can get them out at playtime.

- Take young people to places where they can be active, such as public parks, community sports fields or basketball courts. A stimulating environment and some semi-formal playtime will soon see the children running around a recreation area. With only a small amount of encouragement children will develop their own games and make their own rules.

- Be positive about the physical activities in which the children participate out of school and encourage them to be interested in new activities. If any child has been involved in sporting activities encourage them to share their stories in assembly or through the school website. Make physical activity an aspirational thing to do.

- Make physical activity fun. Fun activities can be either structured or non-structured. Activities can range from team sports or individual sports to recreational activities such as walking, running, skating, bicycling, swimming, playground activities or free-time play.

- Be safe! Always provide protective equipment such as helmets, wrist pads or knee pads and ensure that activities are age appropriate.

> **"Physical fitness is not only one of the most important keys to a healthy body, it is the basis of dynamic and creative intellectual activity."**
> **JF Kennedy**

Let's get going!

Research shows quite clearly that we all need exercise, whether young or old. In the modern world there are more and more labour-saving devices available both inside and outside the home. The result is that we lead a much more sedentary life than our predecessors.

Most of us claim we want to exercise and we know it is good for us but we do not necessarily know how to go about it, how much to do, what kind of exercise to do and how we can judge progress.

Most exercise programmes require special equipment, often only available in a gym, which makes it difficult to exercise every day.

Also, considerable time is often required, which you may not have to spare.

It is therefore obvious that what is needed is a programme which overcomes these obstacles; one which does not require special equipment or long periods of time, and which also is easy to understand, where it is clear what to do next and how to measure your progress. This is such a programme, it requires no specialist equipment, it takes less than 15 minutes a day and needs only a small amount of space.

How it works

As with every other exercise regime, this one begins with easy exercises and gradually progresses in difficulty. As your fitness level improves, so the work load needed increases. This is done in two ways:

- The time taken by each level remains the same throughout, but the number of repeats necessary increases.

- At the same time as you move on from one chart to the next, the difficulty of the exercises gradually increases.

This means that you do the exercises on each chart at every level from one to twelve, but you gradually increase the number of repetitions you do. As you progress from one chart to another, the exercise described has been modified slightly to make it a little more demanding.

It is recommended that you do each exercise in turn. Do not leave any out, and do not try to go faster than is recommended.

The plan is that all the exercises on a chart can be completed within eleven or twelve minutes. It is likely, however, that at first some will take longer than others. This is perfectly normal and acceptable.

Chart 1

Physical capacity rating scale

Level	Exercise					Minutes for:	
	1	2	3	4	5	½ mile run	1 mile walk
A+	20	18	22	13	400	5½	17
A	18	17	20	12	375	5½	17
A–	16	15	18	11	335	5½	17
B+	14	13	16	9	320	6	18
B	12	12	14	8	305	6	18
B–	10	11	12	7	280	6	18
C+	8	9	10	6	260	6½	19
C	7	8	9	5	235	6½	19
C–	6	7	8	4	205	6½	19
D+	4	5	6	3	175	7	20
D	3	4	5	3	145	7½	21
D–	2	3	4	2	100	8	21
Minutes for each exercise	2	1	1	1	6		

Age Groups
6 yrs maintains   Level B
7 yrs maintains   Level A

The meaning of the charts

On the following pages you will find an explanation of what is meant on the chart pages. Check back to the chart above with each paragraph heading.

My progress

Physical capacity rating scale

Level	Exercise					Minutes for:	
	1	2	3	4	5	1 mile run	1 mile walk
A+							
A							
A–							
B+							
B							
B–							
C+							
C							
C–							
D+							
D							
D–							
Minutes for each exercise	2	1	1	1	6		

	Date	Height	Weight
My aim			
Start			
Finish			

Exercise

The numbers used as headings at the top of the charts are the exercises which are numbered 1 to 10. This means that the column with the heading 1 is concerned with exercise 1, etc. Each exercise is illustrated and described on the pages after each chart.

Level

The numbers which run down the left-hand side of the charts refer to the various levels within the programme and each one refers to the line of numbers next to it under the various exercise headings. So, if you look at level 14 you will see that this tells you to carry out exercise 3 seven times, but exercise 6 should be repeated 15 times.

How far should you continue?

The physical level to which you should aim to progress depends upon your age range. The charts are aimed at the average person, so some will be capable of more than others.

Tips to help

- Don't skip a day. The more these exercises become part of your routine, the better you will be and feel.

- You may come across a level which you find very difficult to complete in anything like 11-12 minutes, but keep at it and progress will be seen. You are not competing with anyone else, just against your own body.

- You may find it hard to count all the steps needed in exercise 5. It is easy to lose count. Try dividing the number of steps needed by 75 or 50. On a nearby surface place a row of something, such as coins or buttons, equal to the answer. Do your first set of 75 or 50 steps and move one counter. Repeat until you have moved them all.

How to make a start

It is best if the exercises can be done at the same time each day, so choose a time when you are likely to have 11-12 minutes to spare on a regular basis, perhaps in the early morning, although you may prefer the evening, or some other time, but whatever time you choose, try hard to stick to it *and start today*.

Your progress

The Progress Chart is there to assist you in keeping a record of the progress you are making. Make a note of the starting and finishing date of each level. Also, write down your feelings about each level. Select an achievable aim and write this on the bottom chart in the box labelled 'My Aim'. Your present measurement should be recorded on the start line. When you come to the end of each chart, make a note of your new measurements on the finish line. The changes may be quite subtle as fitness takes time and effort, so the results will not be amazing, but they will be positive. Combine these exercises with a balanced and sensible diet, and you will have success.

Fitness goals

These depend upon your age when starting the programme. Each age group has set a target they should aim to reach. The goals described are average for those taking part in each age group. Your goal then is the level of fitness which is achievable on average for someone of your age, without becoming stressed or over fatigued. As with any other average there will always be those who surpass the average and an equal number who don't quite make it. This is normal.

If you feel you really can go on further than the goals set, go for it, but on the other hand, if you find progress very difficult you need to decide to stop at a level you can maintain.

Sometimes you will reach a plateau with a particular level, but in most cases, if you persist, you will eventually succeed, usually after a few days. The goals are only meant to be guides. If, after a few days, you are not improving, you have almost certainly reached the maximum fitness as far as this exercise programme is concerned.

Caution

If, for some reason, you have a break in the programme for two weeks or more and then decide to restart, it is best to start at a level a little below the one you had reached before you stopped, perhaps even as far back as the previous chart, if you have been ill perhaps. Begin again at a level you find comfortable and then progress from there.

Instructions for following the plan

First choose the goal for your age group. Mark this on the chart. Then note on the chart the minimum number of days you should spend on a level. Do not try to move on faster than the rates of progress recommended.

To begin and to progress

Level 1 starts at the base of Chart 1. Keep at this until you can do it without strain in 11/12 minutes or less. Once you can do this, move on to Level 2, and so on. Move on up the levels and the charts until you reach the level where you feel you have reached your full level of physical fitness or else the level which is the recommended one for your age group.

Once you reach your goal

This may seem a long way away, but you will get there. After this point has been reached you only need to exercise on THREE DAYS EACH WEEK in order to keep up your level of fitness.

Chart 1

If your age in years is	Your goal is (level)	Recommended number of days			
		Chart 1	Chart 2	Chart 3	Chart 4
7-8	30	1	1	2	-
9-10	34	1	1	2	-
11-12	38	1	1	2	3
13-14	41	1	1	2	3
15-17	44	1	1	2	3
18-19	40	1	2	3	4

Chart 1

Physical capacity rating scale

Level	Exercise					Minutes for:	
	1	2	3	4	5	½ mile run	1 mile walk
12	20	18	22	13	400	5½	17
11	18	17	20	12	375	5½	17
10	16	15	18	11	335	5½	17
9	14	13	16	9	320	6	18
8	12	12	14	8	305	6	18
7	10	11	12	7	280	6	18
6	8	9	10	6	260	6½	19
5	7	8	9	5	235	6½	19
4	6	7	8	4	205	6½	19
3	4	5	6	3	175	7	20
2	3	4	5	3	145	7½	21
1	2	3	4	2	100	8	21
Minutes for each exercise	2	1	1	1	6		

Age Groups

6 yrs maintains Level 8

7 yrs maintains Level 11

My progress

Physical capacity rating scale

Level	Exercise					Minutes for:	
	1	2	3	4	5	1 mile run	1 mile walk
12							
11							
10							
9							
8							
7							
6							
5							
4							
3							
2							
1							
Minutes for each exercise	2	1	1	1	6		

	Date	Height	Weight
My aim			
Start			
Finish			

1   Toe touching

Stand with your feet apart and your arms up. Now, bend over so that you can reach the floor with your fingertips and then rise and stretch backwards. Keep your legs straight, but do not strain.

CHART 1

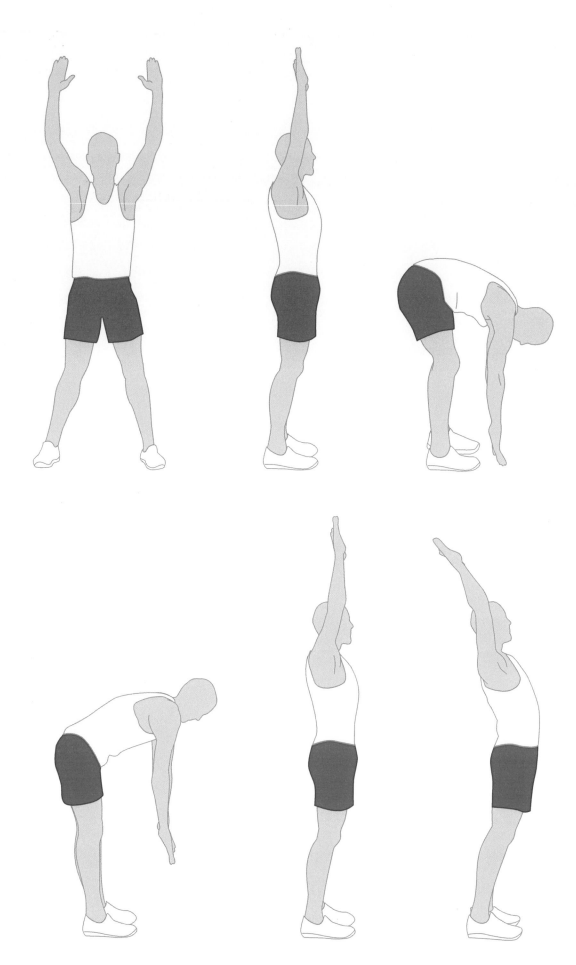

2 Sit-ups

Lie on your back with your arms by your sides and with your feet about six inches apart. Sit up enough to enable you to see your heels. Your legs must remain straight and your head and shoulders must lift up from the floor. Return to the start position.

CHART 1

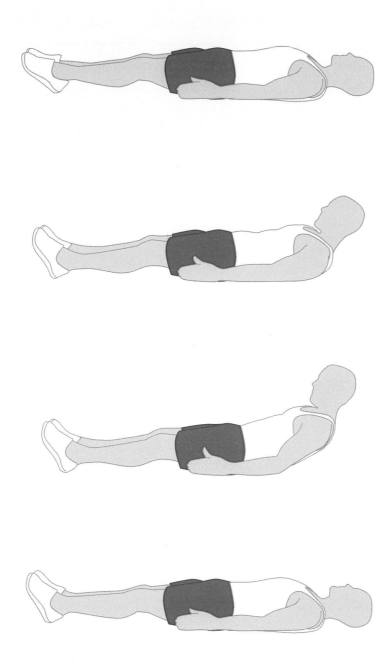

3   Leg raising

Lie on your front with your arms at your sides and with your palms under your thighs. Raise your head together with one leg. Return to the start position. Repeat with the other leg. Count once when the second leg is returned to the floor. Your legs must remain straight and you should lift the leg up so that it is separated from the palm.

CHART 1

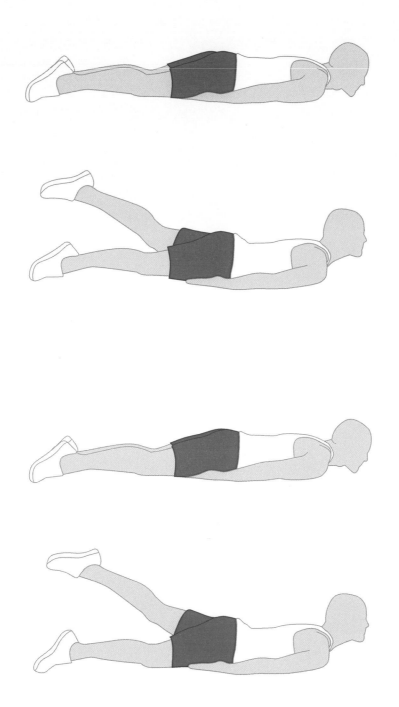

4 Push-ups

Lie on your front with your hands placed under your shoulders and with your palms down on the floor. Keeping your knees on the floor, lift up your upper body by straightening your arms to their full extent. Bend your arms once more to lower yourself to the ground until your chest comes back into contact with the floor.

CHART 1

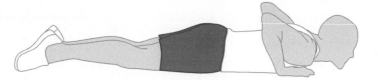

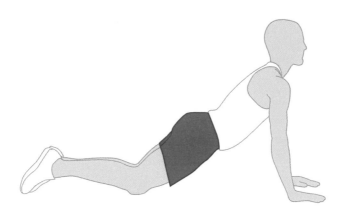

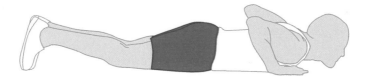

5   The stationary run and scissor steps

You count one step each time your left foot leaves the ground. You need to lift each foot at least 4 inches above the ground. Once you have counted 75 steps, carry out 10 scissor steps.

Scissor steps

Stand with your right leg placed forward and your other leg placed behind you. Your left arm should be extended at shoulder height forwards and with your right one extended behind you. Now jump, reversing these positions.

CHART 1

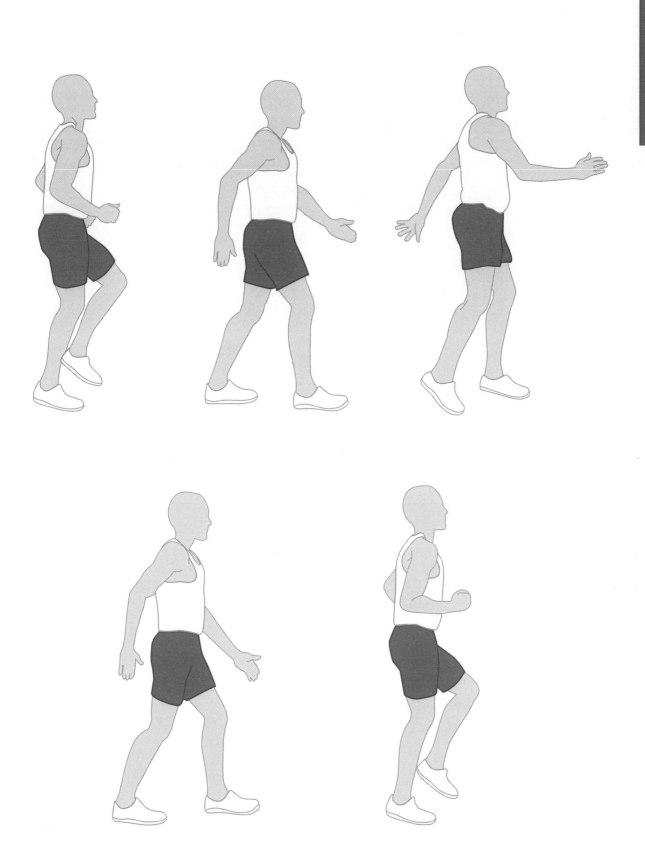

Chart 2

If your age in years is	Your goal is (level)	Recommended number of days			
		Chart 1	Chart 2	Chart 3	Chart 4
7-8	30	1	1	2	-
9-10	34	1	1	2	-
11-12	38	1	1	2	3
13-14	41	1	1	2	3
15-17	44	1	1	2	3
18-19	40	1	2	3	4

Chart 2

Physical capacity rating scale

Level	Exercise					Minutes for:	
	1	2	3	4	5	1 mile run	2 mile walk
24	30	23	33	20	500	9	30
23	29	21	31	19	485	9	31
22	28	20	29	18	470	9	32
21	26	18	27	17	455	9½	33
20	24	17	25	16	445	9½	33
19	22	16	23	15	440	9½	33
18	20	15	21	14	425	10	34
17	19	14	19	13	410	10	34
16	18	13	17	12	395	10	34
15	16	12	15	11	380	10½	35
14	15	11	14	10	360	10½	35
13	14	10	13	9	335	10½	35
Minutes for each exercise	2	1	1	1	6		

Age Groups
8 yrs maintains   Level 13
9 yrs maintains   Level 16
10 yrs maintains Level 19
11 yrs maintains Level 22

My progress

Physical capacity rating scale

Level	Exercise					Minutes for:	
	1	2	3	4	5	1 mile run	2 mile walk
24							
23							
22							
21							
20							
19							
18							
17							
16							
15							
14							
13							
Minutes for each exercise	2	1	1	1	6		

	Date	Height	Weight
My aim			
Start			
Finish			

1   Floor touch and bounce

Stand with your feet astride and with your arms
raised upwards. Bend and touch the floor between
your feet, bounce up part way and then touch
again, before stretching and extending your
back to the rear. Keep your knees as straight
as you can, but do not strain to do so.

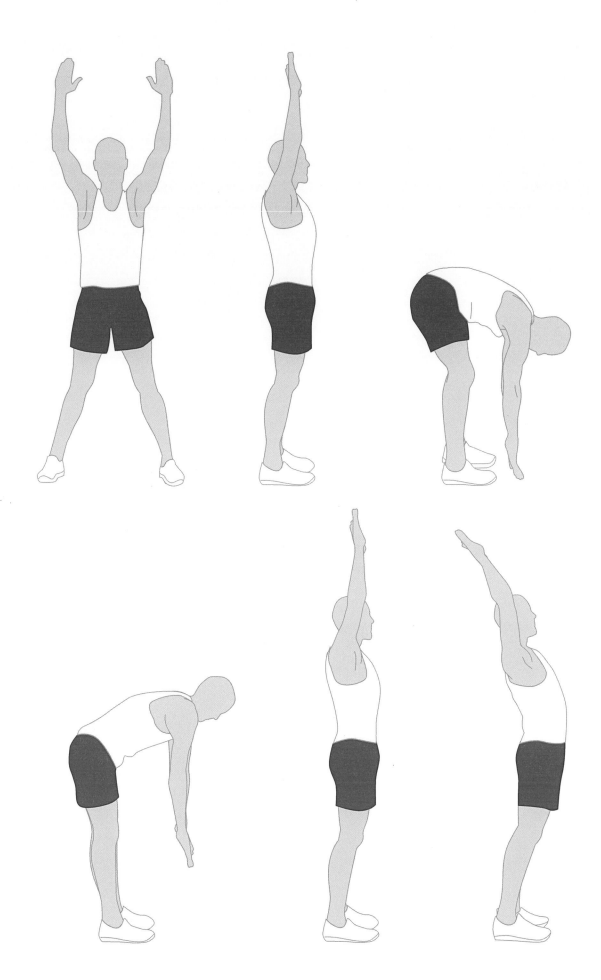

CHART 2

2   Sit-ups

Lie flat on the floor. Your arms should be at your side and your legs straight. Sit up so that your back is now in a vertical position. Keep your feet on the floor. You may find it useful to hook your feet underneath a chair, you should allow your knees to bend a little.

CHART 2

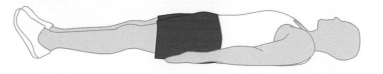

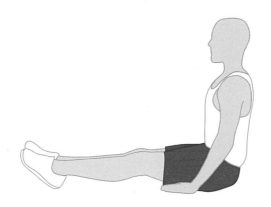

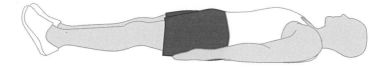

3   Front pull-ups

Lie face down. Your hands should be placed beneath your thighs. Raise your legs together with your head and shoulders. Your legs should remain in a straight position and your thighs should clear your hands.

CHART 2

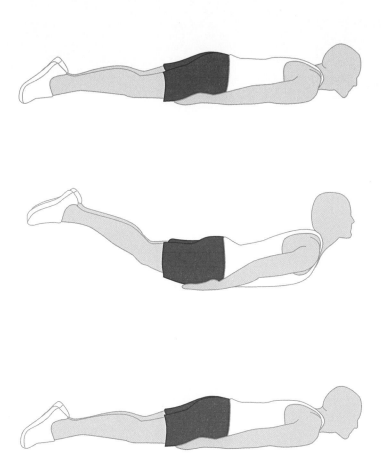

4 Push-ups

Lie face down with your hands placed under your shoulders and with your hands turned so that your palms are in contact with the floor. Push up on your arms to lift your body up from the floor until only your toes and palms are in contact with the floor. You should keep your back in a straight line. Return to the first position so that your chest is in contact with the floor.

CHART 2

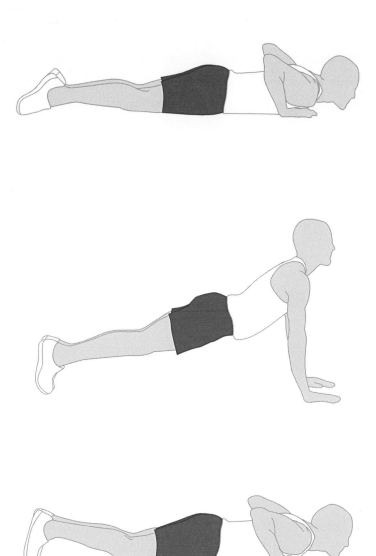

5 Running on the spot and astride jumps

Each time you lift your left foot up from the floor counts as one. Your feet should be lifted at least 4 inches up from the floor. After you have counted to 75, carry out 10 astride jumps.

Astride jumps

Your feet should be placed closely next to each other, and your arms should be placed alongside your sides. Take a jump with your arms held out straight to the sides slightly above the shoulder line. You should land with your feet astride. Jump again back to the start position and count one.

CHART 2

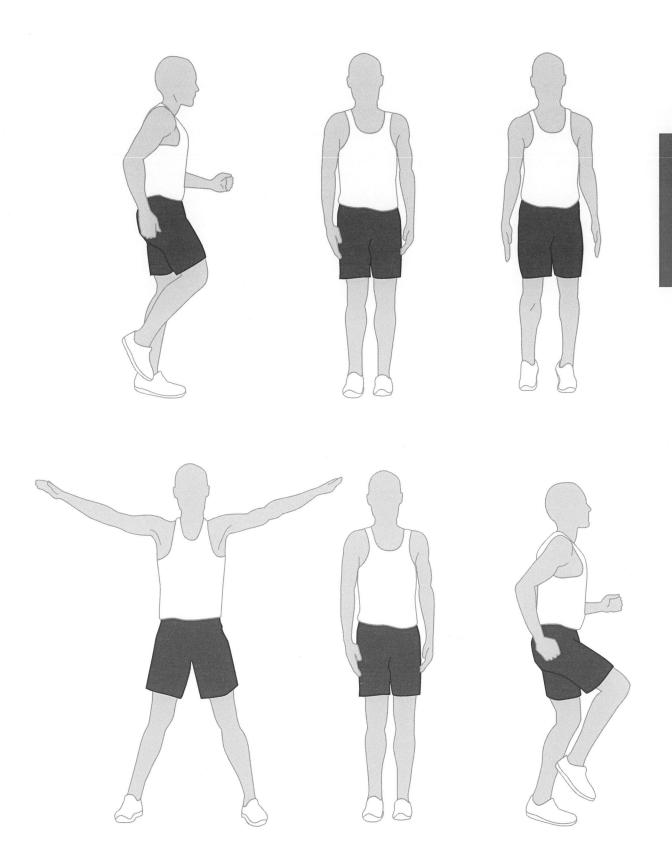

Chart 3

If your age in years is	Your goal is (level)	Recommended number of days			
		Chart 1	Chart 2	Chart 3	Chart 4
7-8	30	1	1	2	-
9-10	34	1	1	2	-
11-12	38	1	1	2	3
13-14	41	1	1	2	3
15-17	44	1	1	2	3
18-19	40	1	2	3	4

Chart 3

Physical capacity rating scale

Level	Exercise					Minutes for:	
	1	2	3	4	5	1 mile run	2 mile walk
36	30	32	47	24	550	8	25
35	30	31	45	22	540	8	25
34	30	30	43	21	525	8	25
33	28	28	41	20	510	8¼	28
32	28	27	39	19	500	8¼	26
31	28	26	37	18	490	8¼	26
30	26	25	35	17	480	8½	27
29	26	24	34	17	465	8½	27
28	26	23	33	16	450	8½	27
27	24	22	31	15	430	8¾	28
26	24	21	30	15	415	8¾	28
25	24	20	29	15	400	8¾	29
Minutes for each exercise	2	1	1	1	6		

Age Groups
12 yrs maintains Level 27
13 yrs maintains Level 30
14 yrs maintains Level 33

My progress

Physical capacity rating scale

Level	Exercise					Minutes for:	
	1	2	3	4	5	1 mile run	2 mile walk
36							
35							
34							
33							
32							
31							
30							
29							
28							
27							
26							
25							
Minutes for each exercise	2	1	1	1	6		

	Date	Height	Weight
My aim			
Start			
Finish			

1   Floor touchdown

You should stand with your arms up and your feet astride. Bend so that you can touch the floor 6 inches to the left of your left foot. Bounce and touch the floor again, this time between your feet and then outside your right foot, before standing up and bending back as far as you can. This counts as one. When you reach the halfway point in your count, reverse your directions, that is touch the right side first. Do not struggle to keep your knees in a straight position.

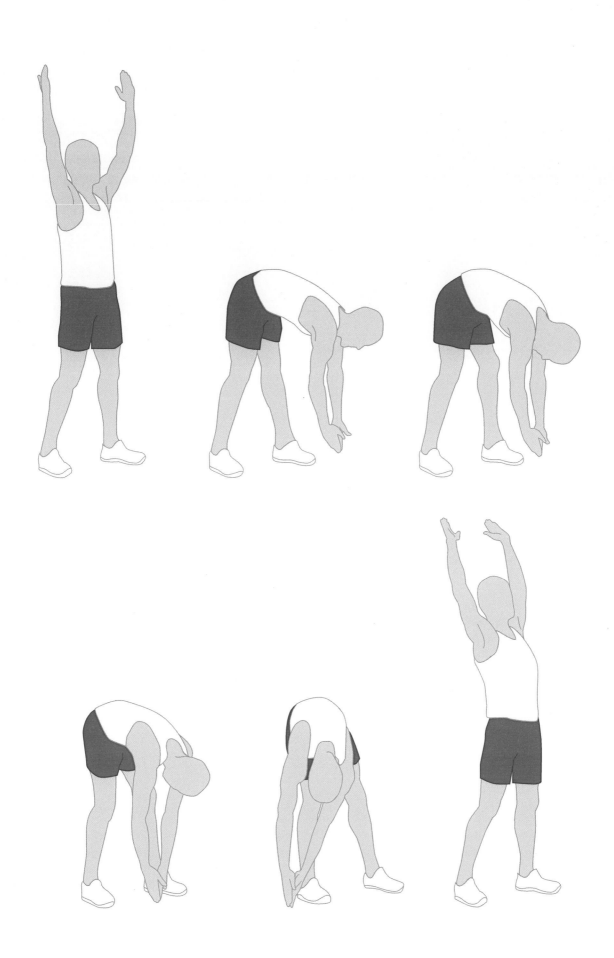

CHART 3

2 Sit–ups

Lie down on your back with your hands clasped at the back of your head. Your legs should be straight and with your heels six inches apart. Keeping your feet on the floor, perhaps hooked below a chair, sit up into the vertical position.

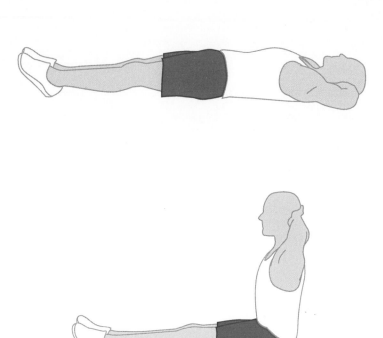

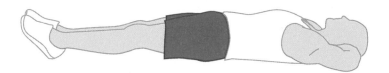

CHART 3

3 Lift-ups

Lie on your front with your hands clasped behind your lower back. Now lift up both your head and upper body, as well as your legs and feet, as far as you can. Your legs should remain straight and your thighs should be raised above the floor. Return to the first position.

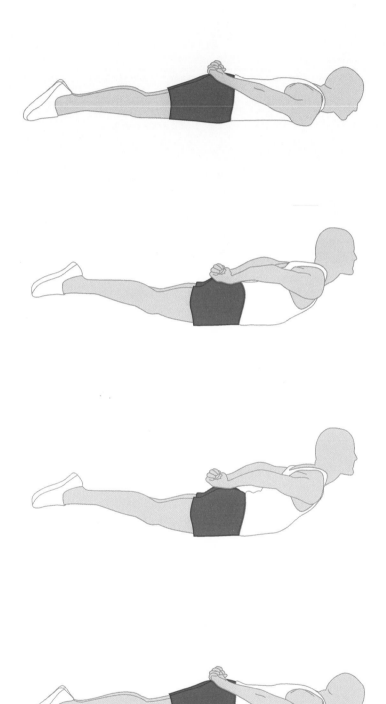

CHART 3

4 Push-ups with touches

Lie on your front with your hands placed under your shoulders and with your palms placed down to touch the floor. Touch the floor with your chin in front of your hands. Next, touch the floor with your brow and then straighten your arms to raise your body. These are three distinct movements which count as one.

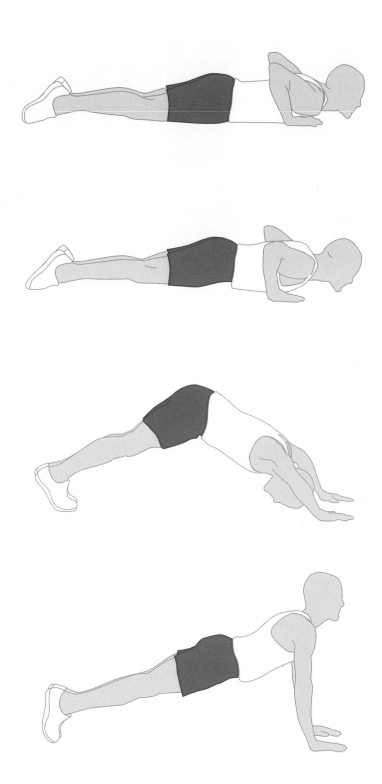

CHART 3

5 Running on the spot and half knee bending

Run on the spot, lifting each foot at least 4 inches up. Each time your left foot returns to the floor you can count one. After a count of 75, carry out 10 half knee bends.

Half knee bending

With your feet placed close together, place your hands on your hips and bend your knees to create an angle of about 110 degrees. Straighten until you are erect, and then lift your heels up from the floor. Your back should remain straight and your feet should not leave contact with the floor. Return to the start position.

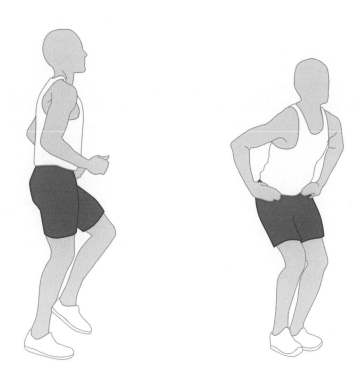

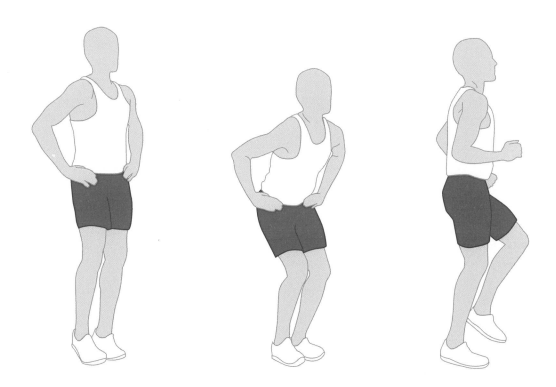

CHART 3

Chart 4

If your age in years is	Your goal is (level)	Recommended number of days			
		Chart 1	Chart 2	Chart 3	Chart 4
7-8	30	1	1	2	-
9-10	34	1	1	2	-
11-12	38	1	1	2	3
13-14	41	1	1	2	3
15-17	44	1	1	2	3
18-19	40	1	2	3	4

Chart 4

Physical capacity rating scale

Level	Exercise					Minutes for:	
	1	2	3	4	5	1 mile run	2 mile walk
48	30	22	50	42	400	7	19
47	30	22	49	40	395	7	19
46	30	22	49	37	390	7	19
45	28	21	47	34	380	7¼	20
44	28	21	46	32	375	7¼	20
43	28	21	46	30	365	7¼	20
42	26	19	44	28	355	7½	21
41	26	19	43	26	345	7½	21
40	26	19	43	24	335	7½	21
39	24	18	41	21	325	7¾	23
38	24	18	40	19	315	7¾	23
37	24	18	40	17	300	7¾	23
Minutes for each exercise	2	1	1	1	6		

Age Groups
15 yrs maintains Level 37
16-17 yrs maintains Level 42
17+ yrs maintains Level 45

My progress

Physical capacity rating scale

Level	Exercise					Minutes for:	
	1	2	3	4	5	1 mile run	2 mile walk
48							
47							
46							
45							
44							
43							
42							
41							
40							
39							
38							
37							
Minutes for each exercise	2	1	1	1	6		

	Date	Height	Weight
My aim			
Start			
Finish			

1 Floor touching with arm circling

Stand with your feet placed widely apart and your arms pointing to the sky. Bend down so that you can touch the floor outside your left foot, followed by touching between your feet and then towards the right. Do not try too hard to keep your knees straight. Stand up and bend yourself backwards. Keep your arms raised and describe a circle. After half your count, reverse the direction of your moves.

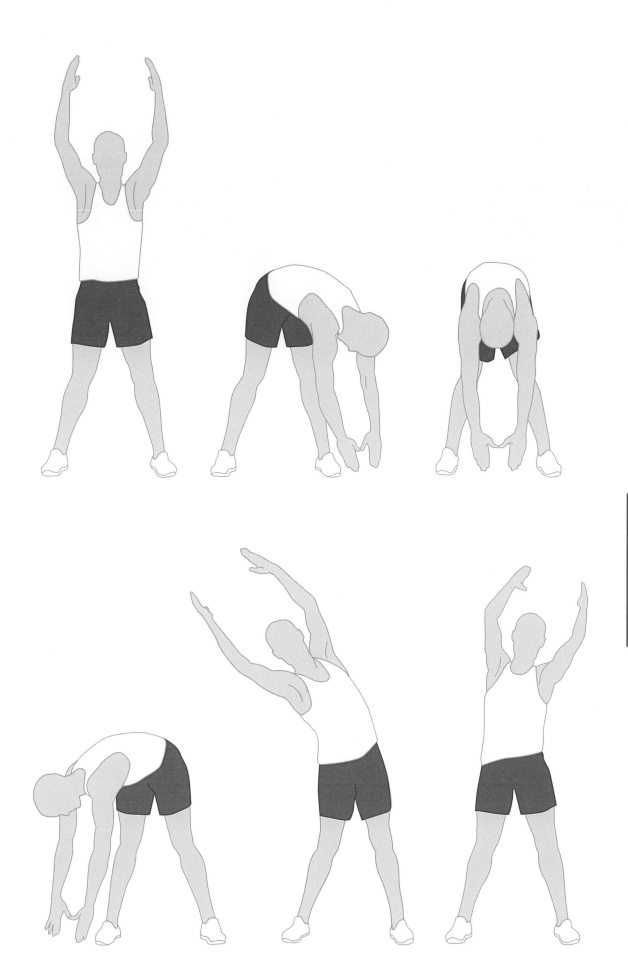

CHART 4

2   Sitting toe touch

You should lie down on your back with your arms back above your head. Your legs should be straight out and your feet close together. Keeping your arms and legs straight, and perhaps hooking your feet under a chair to prevent them rising, sit up so that you can touch your toe tips. Your arms should be kept close to the sides of your head throughout. Lie back down and count one.

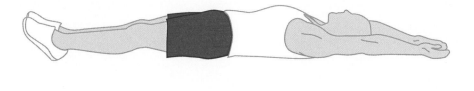

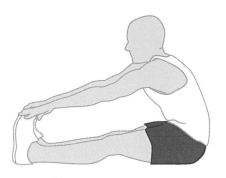

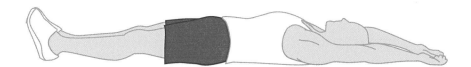

CHART 4

3 Double front lift

Lie down on your front with your arms stretched out to the sides. Your legs should be stretched out and straight. Lift your head, upper body and legs up from the floor as high as you possibly can with arms swinging backwards. Return to the starting position.

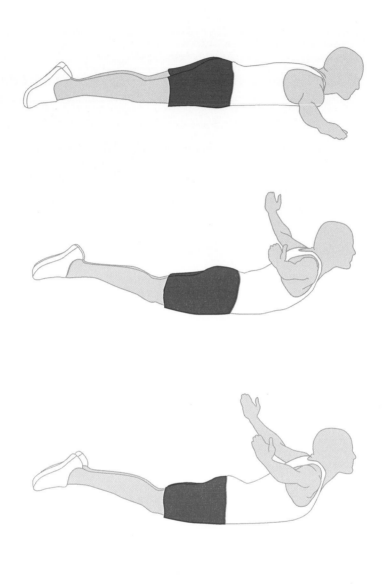

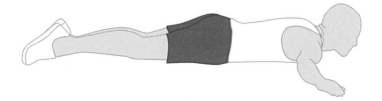

CHART 4

4 Push-ups
from the head

Lie on your front with your hands placed palms down on the floor about a foot each side of your head. Straighten your arms completely to raise your body as high as is possible. Relax and lower yourself until your chest is back in contact with the floor.

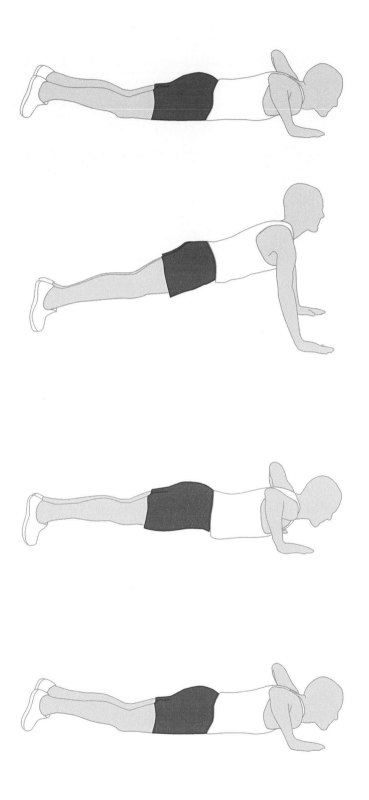

CHART 4

5 Running on the spot with semi-squats

Run on the spot, but this time raise your knees waist high with each step. Do 10 semi-squat jumps after each 75 steps.

Semi-squat jumps

Half crouch with your hands palm down on your knees. Your arms and back should remain as straight as possible. Your feet should be placed so that one foot is slightly ahead of the other. Keeping your body straight, jump up so that your feet are raised above the floor. In the short time before you land, once more reverse the positions of your feet. Crouch again and repeat nine more times.

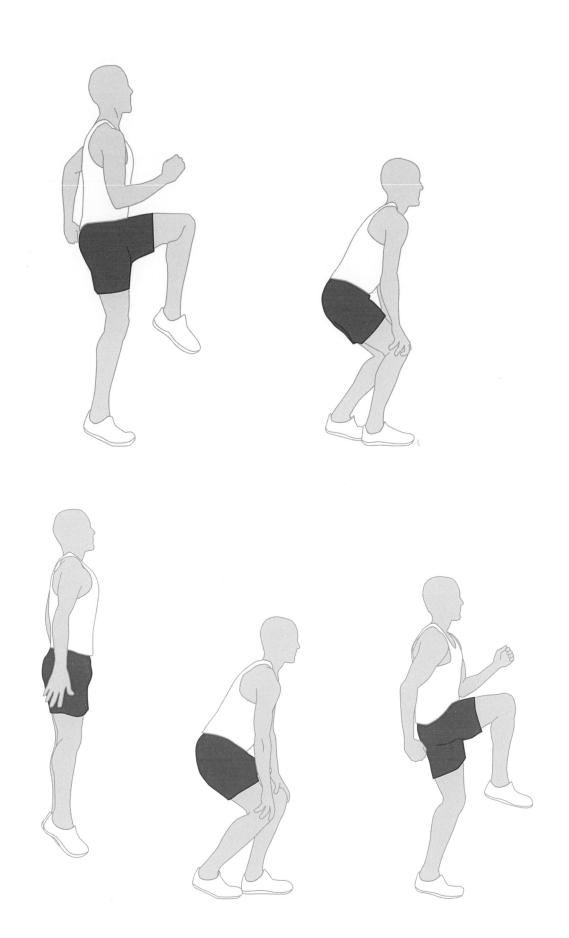

CHART 4

Chart 1

If your age in years is	Your goal is (level)	Recommended number of days			
		Chart 1	Chart 2	Chart 3	Chart 4
7-8	30	1	1	2	-
9-10	34	1	1	2	-
11-12	38	1	1	2	3
13-14	41	1	1	2	3
15-17	44	1	1	2	3

Chart 1

Level	Exercise											
	1	2	3	4	5	6	7	8	9	10	8a	8b
12	9	8	10	40	26	20	30	14	14	170	18	20
11	9	8	10	40	24	18	28	13	14	160	17	18
10	9	8	10	40	22	16	26	12	12	150	16	17
9	7	7	8	36	20	14	24	10	11	140	14	15
8	7	7	8	36	18	12	20	9	10	125	13	14
7	7	7	8	36	16	12	18	8	10	115	11	12
6	5	5	7	28	14	10	16	7	8	100	10	11
5	5	5	7	28	12	8	14	6	6	90	8	9
4	5	5	7	28	10	8	10	5	6	80	7	8
3	3	4	5	24	8	6	8	4	4	70	6	6
2	3	4	5	24	6	4	6	3	3	60	5	5
1	3	4	5	24	4	4	4	3	2	50	4	3
Minutes for each exercise	2				2	1	1	2	1	3	1	1

Recommended number of days at each level ☐

My progress

Level	Start	Finish	Notes
12			
11			
10			
9			
8			
7			
6			
5			
4			
3			
2			
1			

	Date	Height	Weight	Waist	Hips	Bust
My aim						
Start						
Finish						

1 Toe-touching

Start Stand up erect with your feet 12 inches apart and with your arms up above your head.

Bend forward so that you are touching the floor in-between your feet. Don't worry about trying to keep your knees straight.

Return to the first position.

Count Each return to the starting position should be counted as one.

2 Knee raising

Start Stand up straight with your hands by your sides and your feet placed together.

Raise your left knee as high as you possibly can. Grasp your knee and shin and pull your leg in towards your body while keeping your back as straight as possible. Place your foot back on the floor.

Repeat this with your other leg and continue with the legs alternately.

Count A raise of first the left and then the right knee counts as one.

CHART 1

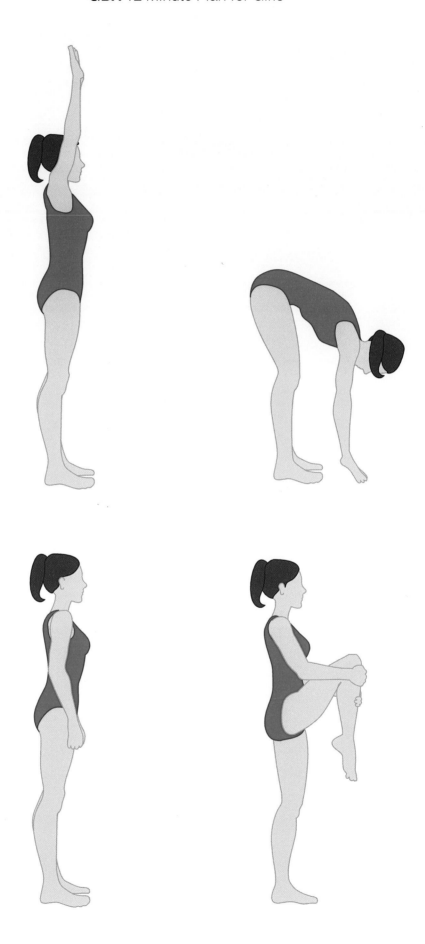

3 Lateral bending

Start Stand up straight with your hands by your sides. Your feet should be about 12 inches apart. While keeping your back straight, bend to the left sideways and slide your hand on that side as far down your leg as possible.

Repeat to the right side.

Count A bend first to the left and then to the right counts as one.

CHART 1

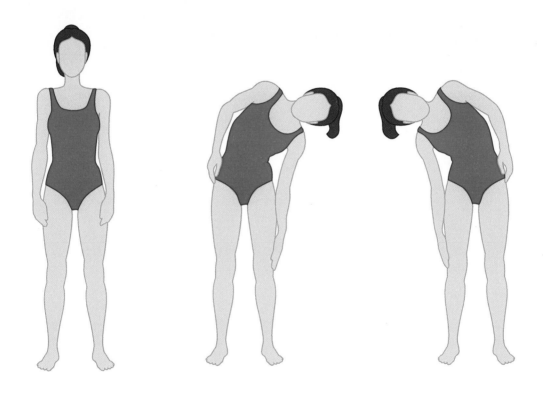

4 Arm circling

Start Stand up straight with your arms at your sides and your feet a foot apart.

Make circles as big as you can with your left arm and then your right one.

Half your total of circles with each arm should be forward and half backwards.

Count A full circle counts as one.

CHART 1

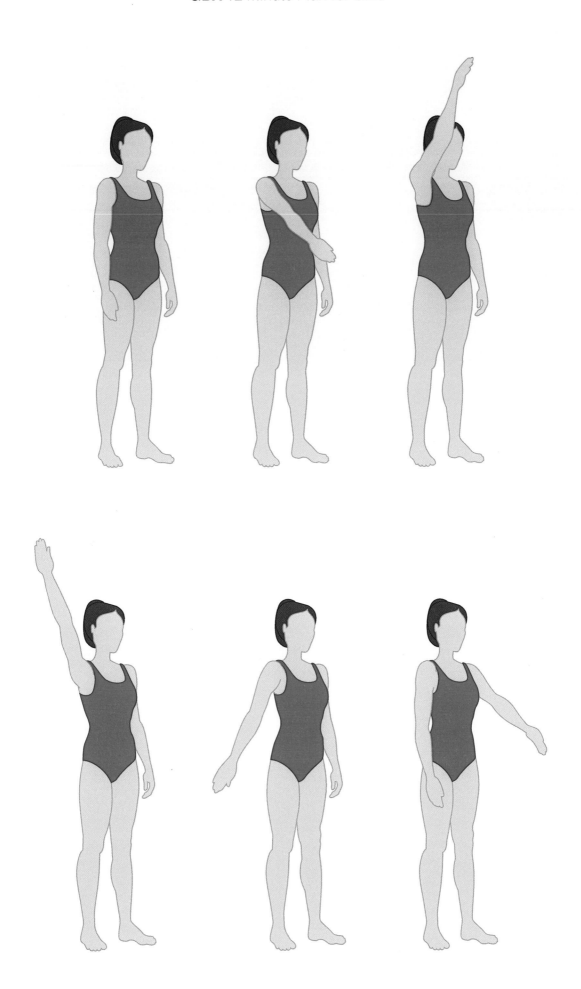

5   Partial sit-ups

Start   Lie down on your back with your arms at your sides and keep your legs straight. Raise your head and shoulder girdle up off the floor until your heels are visible. Lower your head back down.

Count   Each of these partial sit-ups counts as one.

6   Raising the chest and leg raising

Start   Lie face down with your arms along your sides and your hands beneath your thighs and with the palms of your hands pressed along your thighs. Keeping your legs straight, raise your left leg as far as you can and with your head and shoulders raised at the same time. Lower yourself to the floor. Repeat this using the other leg and continue alternating the legs.

Count   Each raise of a leg counts as one.

CHART 1

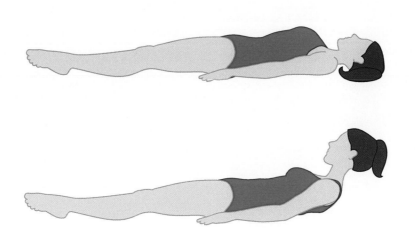

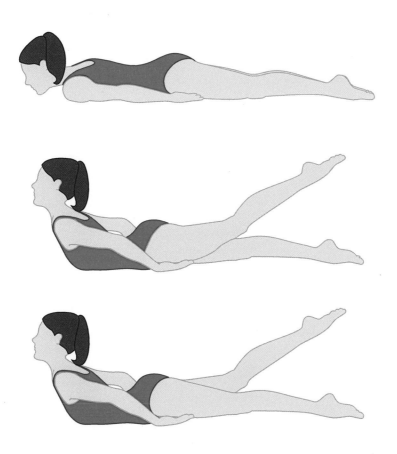

7   Side leg raising

Start   Lie on your side with your legs straight. Your upper arm is used for balance and the lower arm is stretched along the floor above your head. Raise the upper leg about 18-24 inches in the air. Lower it to the start position.

Count   Each raise of a leg counts as one. Do half the required count with one leg and then roll over and use your other leg for the remaining count.

CHART 1

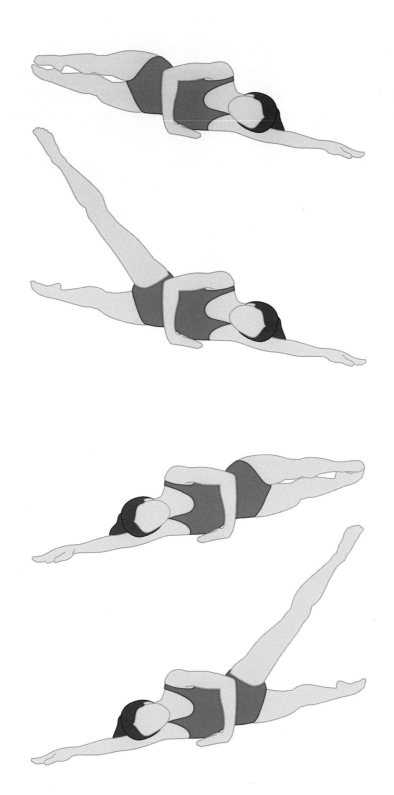

8   Push-ups

Start   Lie with your face down towards the floor. Your legs should be straight and your hands should be placed underneath your shoulders as in the diagram. Keeping your knees and hands in contact with the floor, push your body upwards. Sit back onto your heels. Lower your body back down to the floor.

Count   Each time you lower yourself back down, count one.

CHART 1

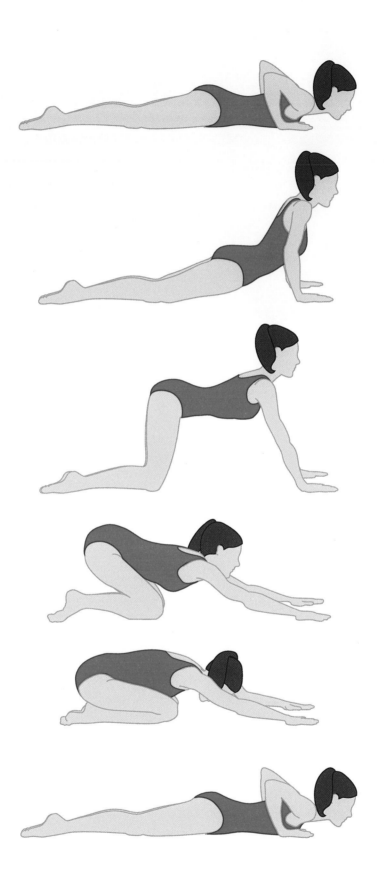

9   Leg lifting

Start   Lie on your back with your arms by your sides and your hands palm side down. Raise your right leg until it is at right angles with the floor, or as near to this as you can possibly do. Lower the leg and repeat with your left leg. Continue, alternating your limbs.

Count   Raising first one leg and then the other counts as one.

CHART 1

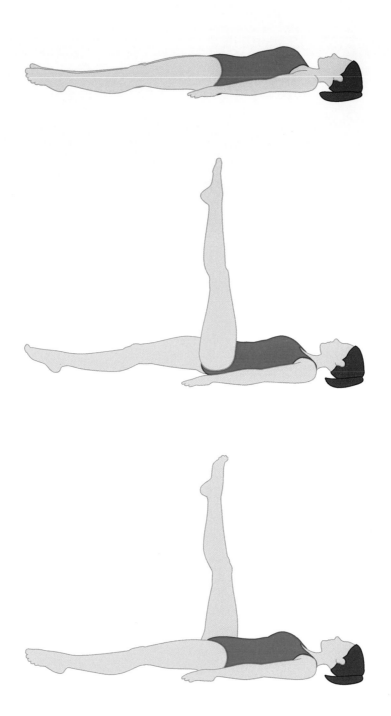

10 Running and hopping

This combines two separate actions

Start Stand up straight with your arms by your sides and your feet placed closely together. Beginning with your left leg, run on the spot. Your feet should be raised at least four inches above the floor with each movement. Don't just move your heels backwards, but also move your knees forwards.

Count Each time you lift your left foot count one. Only these running steps add to your count.

After counting each fifty do ten hops, which means lifting both feet right off the floor together. You should try to raise yourself at least four inches off the floor.

CHART 1

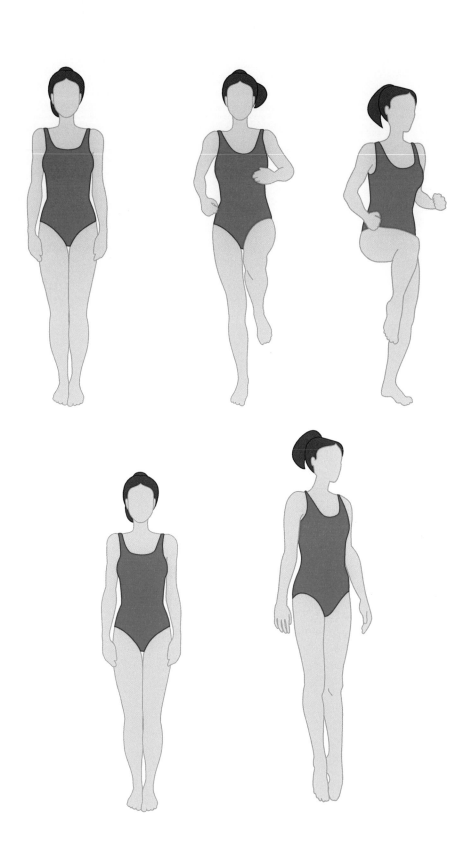

Chart 2

If your age in years is	Your goal is (level)	Recommended number of days			
		Chart 1	Chart 2	Chart 3	Chart 4
7-8	30	1	1	2	-
9-10	34	1	1	2	-
11-12	38	1	1	2	3
13-14	41	1	1	2	3
15-17	44	1	1	2	3

Chart 2

Level	Exercise											
	1	2	3	4	5	6	7	8	9	10	8a	8b
24	15	16	12	30	35	38	50	28	20	210	40	36
23	15	16	12	30	33	36	48	26	18	200	38	34
22	15	16	12	30	31	34	46	24	18	200	36	32
21	13	14	11	26	29	32	44	23	16	190	33	29
20	13	14	11	26	27	31	42	21	16	175	31	27
19	13	14	11	26	24	29	40	20	14	160	28	24
18	12	12	9	20	22	27	38	18	14	150	25	22
17	12	12	9	20	19	24	36	16	12	150	22	20
16	12	12	9	20	16	21	34	14	10	140	19	19
15	10	10	7	18	14	18	32	12	10	130	17	15
14	10	10	7	18	11	15	30	10	8	120	14	13
13	10	10	7	18	9	12	28	8	8	120	12	12
Minutes for each exercise	2				2	1	1	2	1	3	1	1

Recommended number of days at each level ☐

116

My progress

Level	Start	Finish	Notes
24			
23			
22			
21			
20			
19			
18			
17			
16			
15			
14			
13			

	Date	Height	Weight	Waist	Hips	Bust
My aim						
Start						
Finish						

1 Toe-touching

Start   Stand straight with your arms above your head and with your feet a foot apart. Bend forward so that you can touch the floor between your feet. Bob up and then down, repeating the floor-touching once more.

Count   Each time you return to the 'arms above the head position' counts as one.

2 Knee raising

Start   Stand up straight with your feet kept together and with your arms straight at your sides. Raise your left knee as high up as possible. Grasp the knee and the shin with both hands. Pull the leg in towards the body, but keep your back straight. Place your foot back on the floor. Repeat with the other leg and continue alternating the legs used.

Count   Raising first one knee and then the other counts as one.

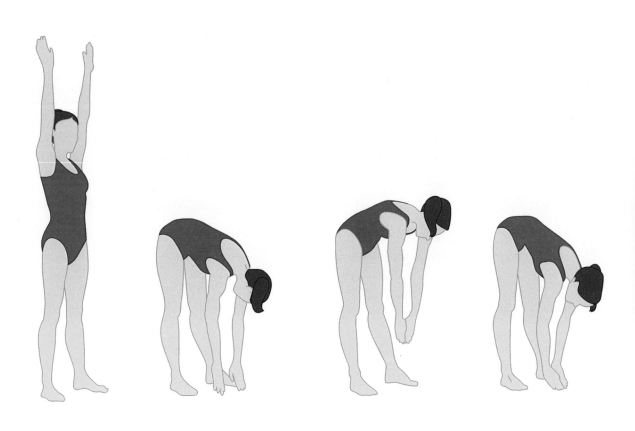

CHART 2

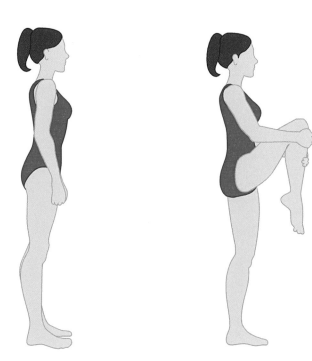

3   Lateral bending

Start   Stand straight with your arms by your sides and your feet placed a foot apart. Keeping your back as straight as possible, bend from waist level to the left side, while sliding your left hand as far down the outer side of the leg as possible. Bob up a few inches and then bend once more. Return to your starting stance and repeat on the alternate side. Continue with a bend to each side in turn.

Count   A bend first to the left and then to the right counts as one.

4   Arm circling

Start   Stand straight with your arms at your sides and your feet placed a foot apart. Using both arms at the same time, make as large backwards circles as you possibly can. After you have done half the number of repetitions required, then change over to forward circles.

Count   Each complete circle counts as one.

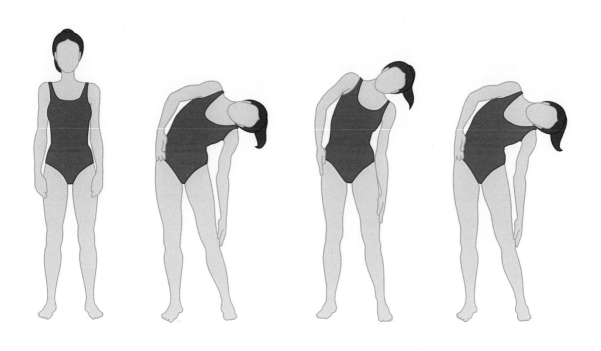

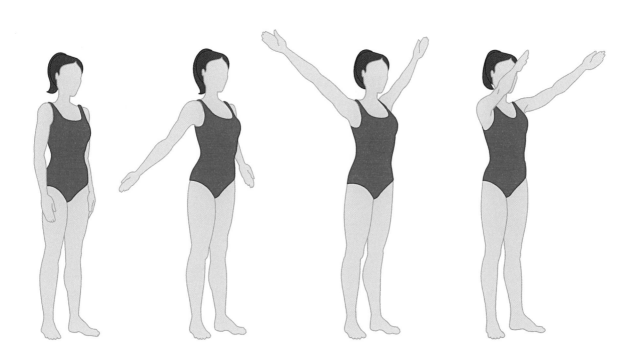

CHART 2

5   Rocking sit-ups

Start   Lie down on your back with your arms over your head. Your knees should be bent so that the soles of your feet are flat on the floor. Swing your arms forward while, at the same time, thrusting your feet forward, moving into a sitting position. Now stretch forward and touch the tips of your toes with your fingers. Go back to the start position.

Count   Every time you return to your starting position, you count one.

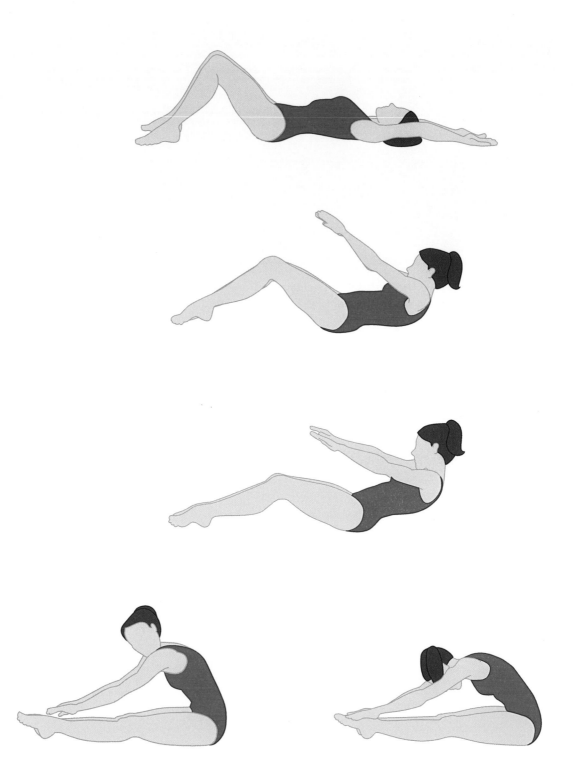

CHART 2

6 Leg and chest raising

Start Lie on your front with your arms at your sides, and your hands should have their palms pressing on the thighs. Keep your legs straight while raising your legs, together with your head and shoulders, as far upwards as possible. Relax and go back to your original position.

Count Each time you return to your starting pose, count one.

7 Side leg raising

Start Lie on your side. You should keep your legs straight and you should have your lower arm stretched above your head. You use the other arm to improve your balance. Raise your upper leg until it is at right angles with the floor, or as near to this as you can manage. Bring your leg back down.

Count Each time you lift your leg up, count one. For half of the required count use your left leg, and then roll over and use the other leg for the rest of the count.

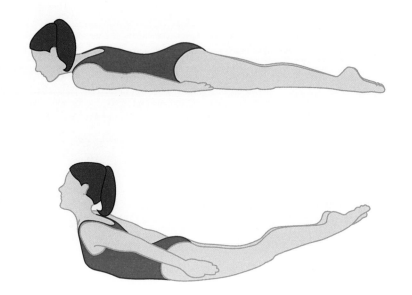

CHART 2

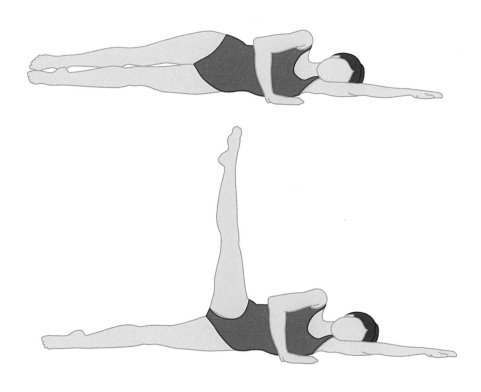

8   Knee push-ups

Start   Begin by lying face down on the floor with your hands placed under your shoulders and your legs kept straight and close together. Push down with your hands until your arms are straight and your torso is off the floor. Your knees should remain in touch with the floor throughout. You should aim to keep your body in as straight a line as possible. Let yourself return to the starting position.

Count   Each return to the flat position counts as one.

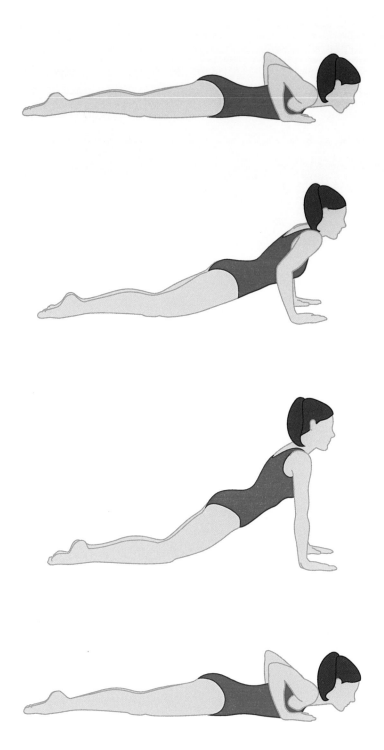

CHART 2

9   Leg overs

Start   Lie on your back with your arms stretched out sideways and your legs straight and together. Raise your right leg to the upright position and then drop it down across your body, as if trying to touch your fingers with the tips of your toes. Raise your leg up again and then return it to the starting position. Repeat this action with your other leg. Your shoulders should stay in contact with the floor and your body should be as straight as possible all the time, and so should your leg.

Count   Each time you return to the first position counts as one.

CHART 2

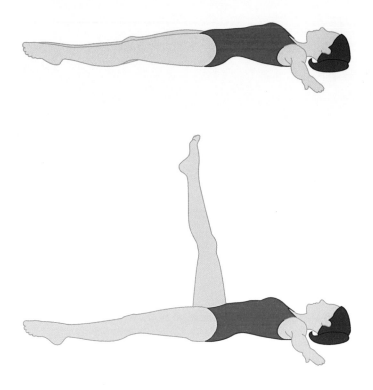

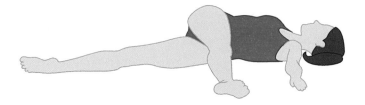

10 Running and stride jumping

Start   Stand straight up with your feet placed together and with your hands placed by your sides. Beginning with your left leg, followed by the right, raise each foot at least four inches from the ground.

Count   Each time your left foot is raised up, this counts as one.

After a count of 50, carry out 10 stride jumps. These begin with your hands at your sides and with your feet together. Jump so that the feet, when you land, are about 18 inches apart. When you jump, raise up your arms to the sides to the height of your shoulders. Then jump again so that your feet come together again and your arms are back at your sides. These two jumps together count as one.

CHART 2

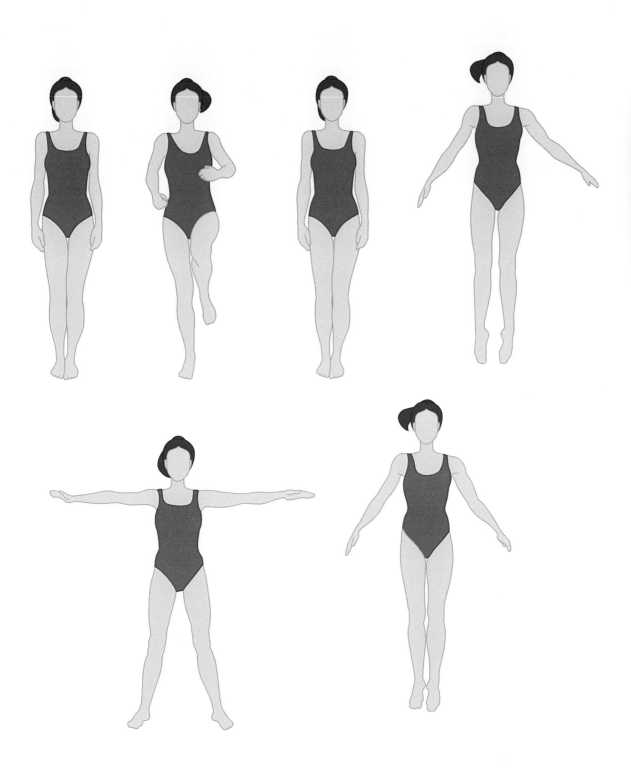

Chart 3

If your age in years is	Your goal is (level)	Recommended number of days			
		Chart 1	Chart 2	Chart 3	Chart 4
7-8	30	1	1	2	-
9-10	34	1	1	2	-
11-12	38	1	1	2	3
13-14	41	1	1	2	3
15-17	44	1	1	2	3

Chart 3

Level	Exercise											
	1	2	3	4	5	6	7	8	9	10	8a	8b
36	15	22	18	40	42	40	60	40	20	240	32	38
35	15	22	18	40	41	39	60	39	20	230	30	36
34	15	22	18	40	40	38	58	37	19	220	29	34
33	13	20	16	36	39	36	58	35	19	210	27	33
32	13	20	16	36	37	36	56	34	18	200	25	31
31	13	20	16	36	35	34	56	32	16	200	24	30
30	12	18	14	30	33	33	54	30	15	190	23	28
29	12	18	14	30	32	31	54	29	14	180	21	26
28	12	18	14	30	31	30	52	27	12	170	20	25
27	10	16	12	24	29	30	52	25	11	160	19	23
26	10	16	12	24	27	29	50	23	9	150	17	21
25	10	16	12	24	26	28	48	22	8	140	16	20
Minutes for each exercise	2				2	1	1	2	1	3	1	1

Age Groups

7-8 yrs maintains Level 30

9-10 yrs maintains Level 34

Recommended number of days at each level ☐

134

My progress

Level	Start	Final	Notes
36			
35			
34			
33			
32			
31			
30			
29			
28			
27			
26			
25			

	Date	Height	Weight	Waist	Hips	Bust
My aim						
Start						
Final						

1   Toe–touching

Start   Stand straight with your feet placed so that they are about 16 inches apart. Bend over and touch the floor to the left of your left foot with both hands; bob up and then back down to touch the floor between your feet; bob again and then touch the floor on the outside of your right foot. Stand up straight again in your starting position.

Count   Each time you stand up straight again counts as one.

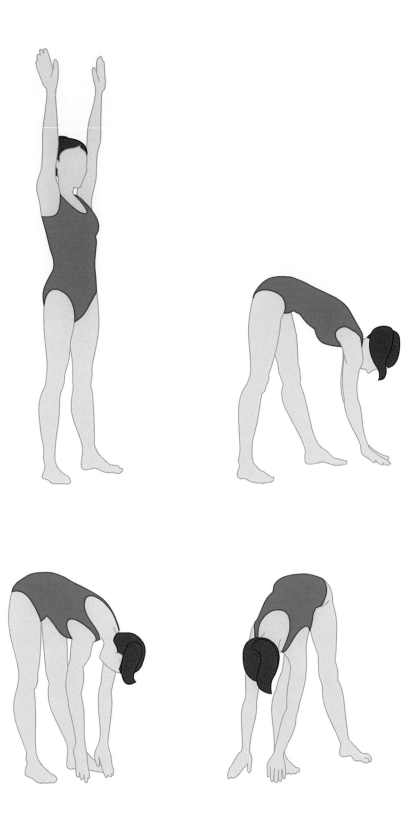

CHART 3

2 Knee raising

Start Stand straight with your feet placed together and with your hands by your sides. Raise your left knee as high as possible and then grasp it, and your shin, with your hands and then draw it close to your body. With your back kept straight, lower your foot to the floor. Now repeat this action with your other knee. Continue to the required count, alternating the legs.

Count Raising first the left and then the right leg counts as one.

3 Lateral bending

Start Stand straight up with your right arm lifted up and over the head, but keep your elbow bent. Your feet should be a foot apart. Keeping your spine straight, bend from the waist to the left side. Press towards the left with your right arm, while at the same time sliding your left hand as far down on your leg as possible. Return to your first position and then change over your arm positions before continuing to the right side. Return to the beginning.

Count A bend first to the left and then to the right counts as one.

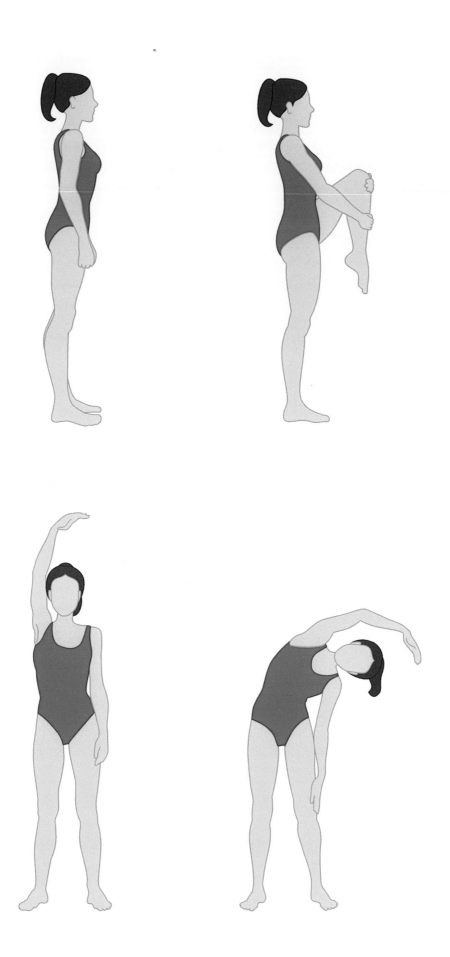

CHART 3

4 Arm circling

Start   Begin by standing up straight with your arms by your sides and your feet placed about a foot apart. Use both arms to make large circles with one arm following the other in a windmill pattern. Half the required number of repetitions should be carried out moving forward and half by swinging the arms backwards.

Count   A full circle of both arms makes a count of one.

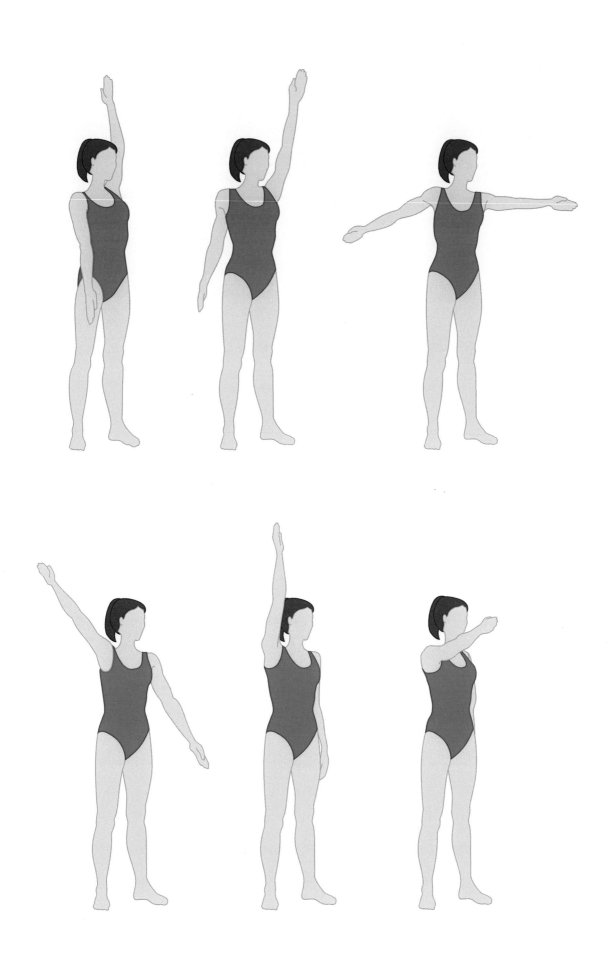

CHART 3

5   Sit-ups

Start   Lie flat on your back with your legs placed together and straight, and with your arms close by your sides. While keeping your back as straight as you possibly can, raise yourself to the sitting position. Slide both hands along your legs towards your toes and touch them. Return to the original position.

Count   Each time you lie back down counts as one.

6   Chest and leg raising

Start   Lie down on your front with your arms stretched out to the sides at shoulder level. Your legs should be placed together and straight. Lift up your whole upper body, together with your legs, which should be as straight as possible. Return to the initial position.

Count   Each return to the first position counts as one.

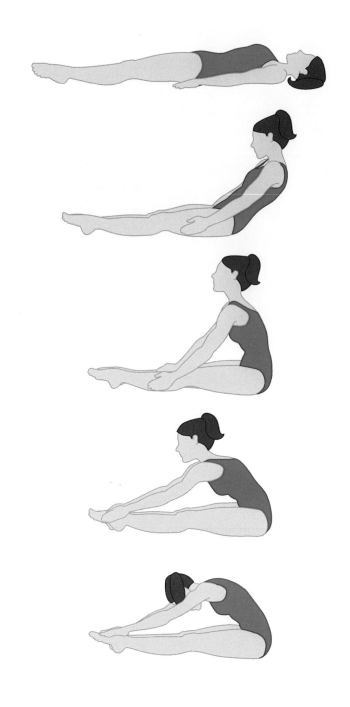

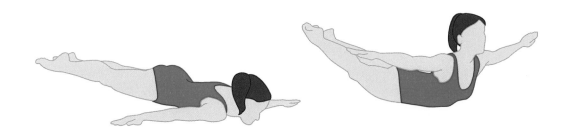

CHART 3

7   Side leg raising

Start   Lie on your side with your legs straight. Your upper arm should be used to give you balance while your lower arm is placed above your head on the floor. Lift up your upper leg until it is at right angles with the floor. Lower the leg to its original position. Do half the number of counts with one leg and the rest with the other.

Count   Each time you raise your leg, count one.

8   Elbow push-ups

Start   Lie down facing the floor. Keep your legs together and straight. Your elbows should be straight under your shoulders, so that they are at right angles to the floor. Keep your head raised throughout. Your forearms should be placed along the floor and your hands should be clasped together. Lift your body up from the floor, keeping it as straight as you can. When you are in the raised position, your body will maintain a straight line and your toes, elbows and forearms keep in contact with the floor surface. Now lower yourself to the original position.

Count   Count one each time you return to the lower position.

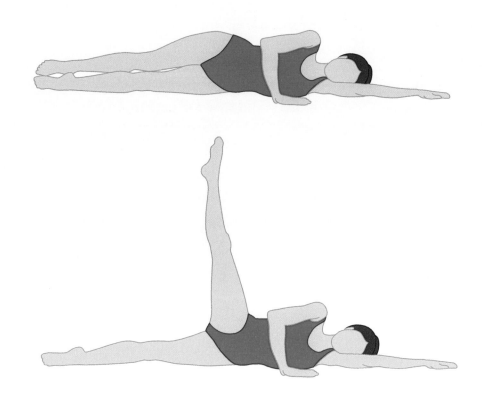

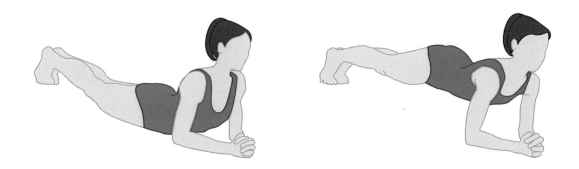

CHART 3

9 Legs over with tuck

Start   Lie on your back with your arms stretched out sideways and with the palms pointing downwards. Your legs should be straightened and kept together. Lift up both your legs towards your body into a tuck position. With your shoulders kept in contact with the floor, lower your legs first to the left, and then to the right. The legs should remain in the tuck position. Return your knees to the starting perpendicular position.

Count   Each time you return to the beginning counts as one.

10 Run and half knee bends

Start   Stand up straight with your arms by your sides and your legs placed together. Beginning with your left foot, raise each foot in turn, lifting them at least 6 inches up from the floor.

Count   Each time your left foot touches the floor counts as one.

After each fifty counts do ten half knee bends.

Half knee bends

Half knee bends start with hands on hips, feet together, body erect. Bend at knees and hips, lowering body until thigh and calf form an angle of about 110 degrees. Do not bend knees past a right angle. Keep back straight. Return to starting position.

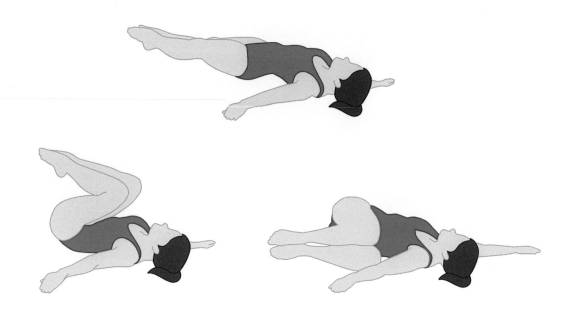

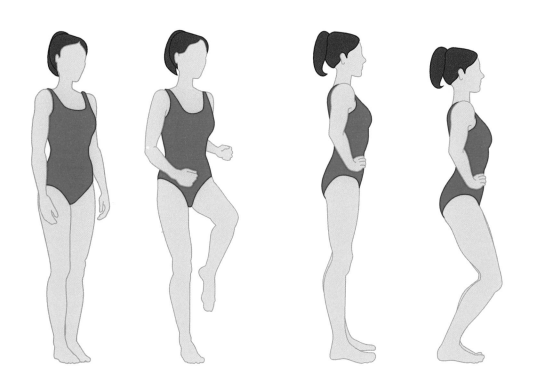

CHART 3

Chart 4

If your age in years is	Your goal is (level)	Recommended number of days			
		Chart 1	Chart 2	Chart 3	Chart 4
7-8	30	1	1	2	-
9-10	34	1	1	2	-
11-12	38	1	1	2	3
13-14	41	1	1	2	3
15-17	44	1	1	2	3

Chart 4

Level	Exercise										
	1	2	3	4	5	6	7	8	9	10	
48	15	26	15	32	48	46	58	30	16	230	
47	15	26	15	32	45	45	56	27	15	220	
46	15	26	15	32	44	44	54	24	14	210	
45	13	24	14	30	42	43	52	21	13	200	
44	13	24	14	30	40	42	50	19	13	190	
43	13	24	14	30	38	40	48	16	12	175	
42	12	22	12	28	35	39	46	13	10	160	
41	12	22	12	28	32	38	44	11	9	150	
40	12	22	12	28	30	38	40	9	8	140	
39	10	20	10	26	29	36	38	8	7	130	
38	10	20	10	26	27	35	36	7	6	115	
37	10	20	10	26	25	34	34	6	5	100	
Minutes for each exercise	2				2	1	1	2	1	3	

Age Groups

11-12 yrs maintains Level 38

13-14 yrs maintains Level 41

15-17 yrs maintains Level 44

17+ yrs maintains Level 48

Recommended number of days at each level ☐

My progress

Level	Start	Final	Notes
48			
47			
46			
45			
44			
43			
42			
41			
40			
39			
38			
37			

	Date	Height	Weight	Waist	Hips	Bust
My aim						
Start						
Final						

1 Toe-touching

Start   Stand upright with your hands over your head and with your feet about 16 inches apart. Bend down to touch the floor to the left of your left foot. Bob up and then touch the floor between your two feet. Bob up again and then touch the floor between the feet once more. Bob up and then bend so that you can touch the floor on the right of your right foot. Return to the upright position.

Count   Count one each time you return to the upright position.

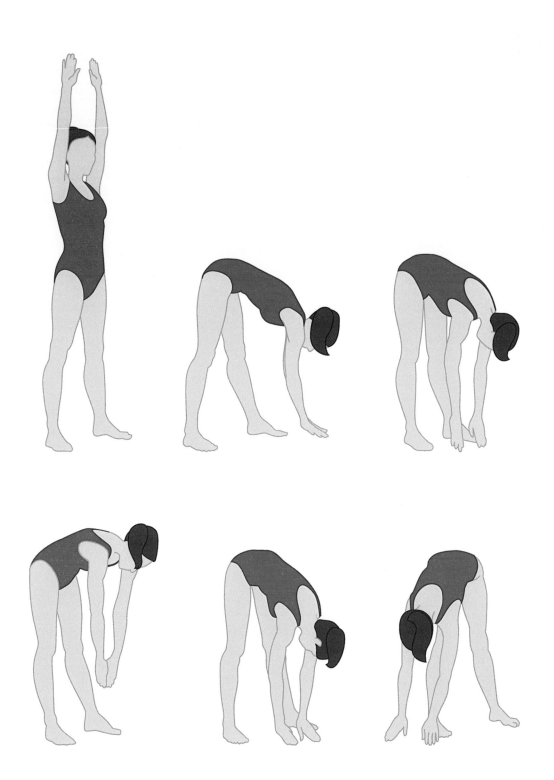

CHART 4

2 Knee raising

Start   Stand upright with your feet together and with your hands by your sides. Lift your left knee as high as you can, holding your knee and shin with your hands. Keep your back straight, while pulling the knee in towards the body. Place the foot back on the floor. Do this with the other leg. Continue to alternate the legs until you reach the required number.

Count   One raising of both knees, one after the other, counts as one.

3 Lateral bending

Start   Stand straight up with your feet a foot apart. Extend your hand over your head with the arm bent at the elbow. Keep your back straight while bending sideways from the waist towards the left. Slide your left hand gradually as far as you can while also pressing to the left with your right hand. Bob a few inches towards the upright and then press to the left once more. Return to the original position and swap over the position of your arms. Repeat on the right side. Alternate from right to left as many times as needed.

Count   One set of bends to the left and right counts as one.

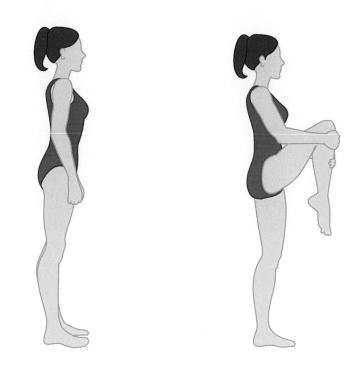

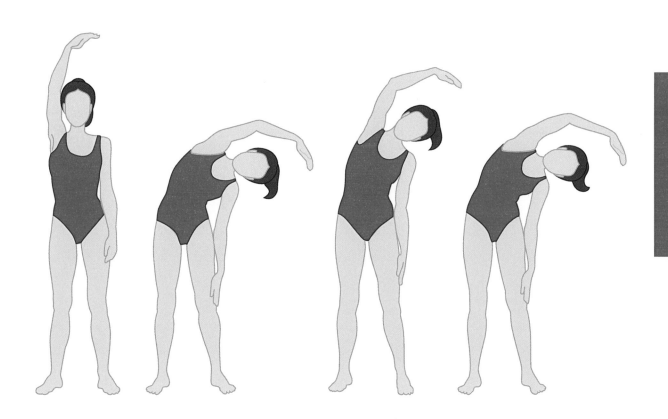

CHART 4

4   Arm flinging

Start   Stand up straight with your feet a foot apart. Your upper arms should be at shoulder height, extended, but with the elbows bent and your fingertips touching in front of you. Do not let your elbows drop while you press them backwards and upwards. Bring your arms back to the first position and then fling your arms out and back and up as far as you can. Go back to the first position.

Count   After each arm fling, count one.

5   Sit-ups

Start   Lie on your back with your legs together and lying straight, and place your hands under your head. Move into a sitting position while keeping your feet on the floor and your back straight. Lower the body back onto the floor.

Count   Each time you lie back down, count one.

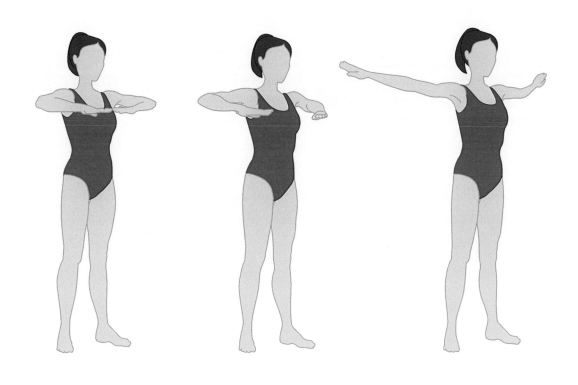

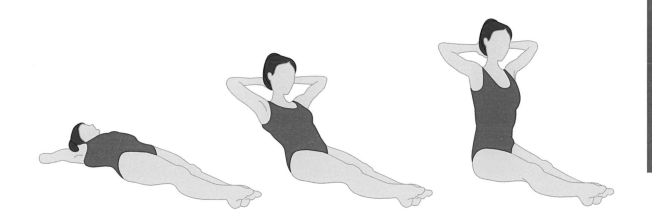

CHART 4

6   Raising the chest and legs

Start   Lie down facing the floor with your hands behind your head and your legs together and straight. Lift up your legs and upper body as far off the floor as you can while you keep your legs in a straight position. Return to the initial position.

Count   Each time you return to the first position, count one.

7   Side leg raising

Start   With your right side in contact with the floor and with your arm straight, support your body weight on the side of your foot and your hand. You may need to use your other hand to give you extra balance. Raise your left leg to a position where it is parallel to the floor surface. Lower the leg once more. Repeat for half the count and then swap sides and do the other half.

Count   Each leg raise and return counts as one.

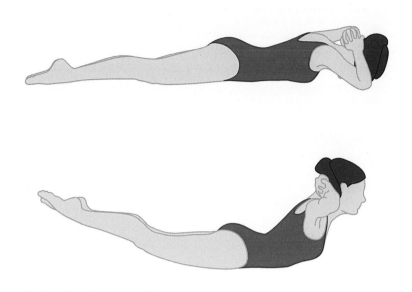

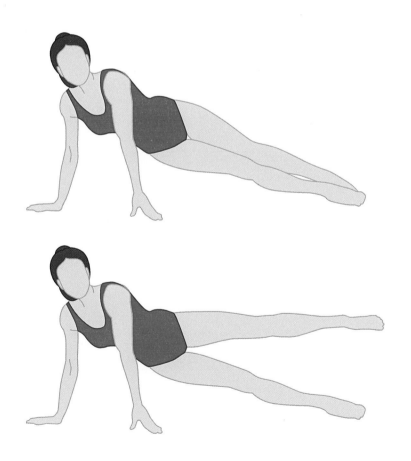

CHART 4

8   Push-ups

Start   Lie on your front. Keep your legs together and straight, but with your toes turned under and with your hands directly underneath your shoulders. Push upwards with the toes and hands until your arms are straight and fully extended. Still keeping your legs and body in one straight line, lower yourself until your chest touches the ground once more.

Count   Each time you return your chest to the floor counts as one.

9   Straight leg overs

Start   Begin by lying down on your back with your arms stretched out to the sides and your palms pointing down to the floor. Your legs should be together and kept straight. Lift both legs until they are at right angles with the floor, at the same time keeping them straight and close together. Lower your legs to the left side, trying to reach your left hand with your toes and twisting from the waist. Lift your legs to the perpendicular position once more and then over to the right. Lift them back up to the upright and then lower them to the starting position.

Count   Each time you place your legs back on the floor, count one.

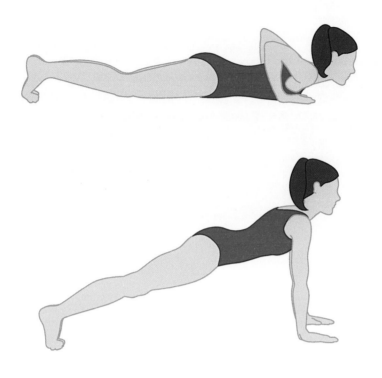

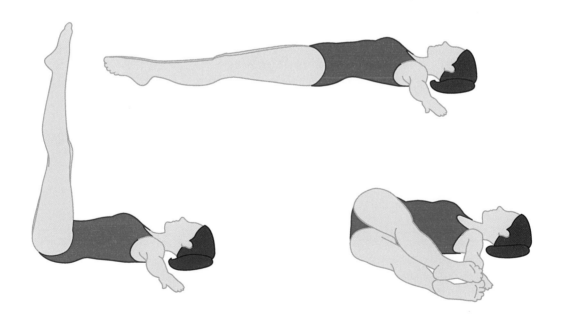

CHART 4

10 Run with semi-squat jumps

Start Stand up straight with your arms by your sides and with your feet placed closely together. Beginning with your left foot, run on the spot, lifting your leg at least 6 inches above the floor.

Count Every time your left foot returns to the floor counts as one.

After you have counted to 50 carry out 10 semi-squat jumps. These are done by dropping into a half crouch with your arms kept straight and with your hands placed on your knees. One foot should be placed just in front of the other and your back should remain as straight as is possible. Jump up into an upright position so that your feet leave the floor and your back is straight. Before you land once more, reverse the position of your two feet. Go back into the crouch position and repeat for a count of ten.

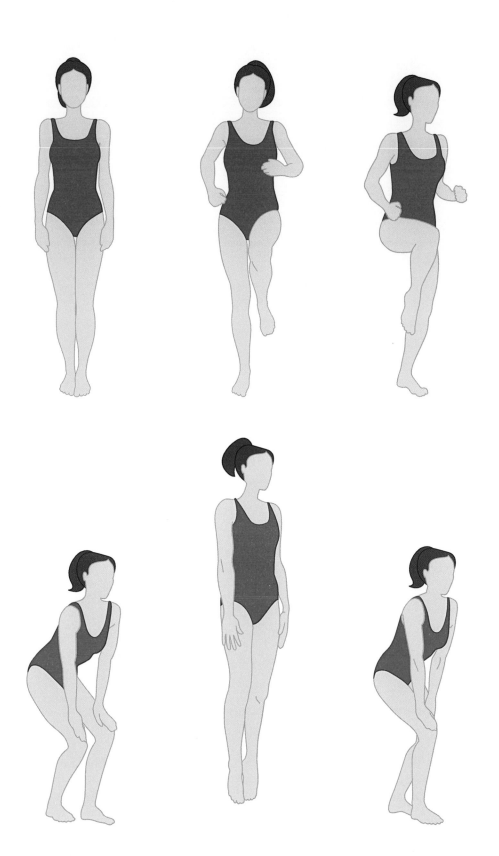

CHART 4